Medicine Under Sail

Medicine Under Sail

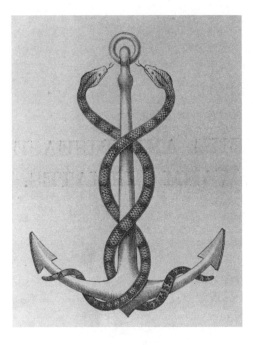

Zachary B. Friedenberg

Naval Institute Press
ANNAPOLIS, MARYLAND

* * *

Naval Institute Press
291 Wood Road
Annapolis, MD 21402

Library of Congress Cataloging-in-Publication Data

Friedenberg, Zachary.
   Medicine under sail / Zachary B. Friedenberg.
   p. cm.
   Includes bibliographical references and index.
   ISBN 1-55750-297-8 (alk. paper)
   1. Medicine, Naval—History. 2. Ship physicians—History. 3. Voyages and travels—Miscellanea. I. Title.
   RC986.F754 2002
   616.9'8024'09—dc21

                                                2001044670

Printed in the United States of America on acid-free paper ∞

09 08 07 06 05 04 03 02   9 8 7 6 5 4 3 2
First printing

Title page photo reprinted from Davidson, *Hygiene and Diseases of Warm Climates*, 1793

Distributed internationally by
Chatham Publishing, 99 High Street, Rochester,
Kent ME1 1LX United Kingdom

Contents

Preface

A Solitary sail that rises
White in the blue mist on the foam.
What is it in far lands, it prizes?
What does it leave behind at home?
Mikhail Lermontov (1814–41)

WHEN THE TRIREME exchanged its oars for sails, when the astronomers introduced celestial navigation, and the compass, astrolabe, and octant freed sailors from the need to follow the coast, seafarers could reach for distant lands—sometimes fabled, sometimes real. The world suddenly expanded, and continents and islands were added to the map that equaled or exceeded the land masses from which the ships departed.

Cartographers replaced sea serpents and mermaids on their maps with defined coasts, harbors, and islands. Shipwrights and sail-makers made faster and more seaworthy vessels and contributed to the ever-increasing waves of exploration and commerce. But the ability of human beings to adjust to months at sea had not been tested, and the health consequences were first unforeseen and then neglected. They presented frustrating impediments to ambition; they kept ships tethered to frequent landfalls. Ships left port with banners flying, urged on by cheering crowds wharfside, to return with the remnants of a crew—hardly able to set a sail, haggard and sick, who had to be carried ashore.

Never considered was the part of the equation that regarded the needs of the human body and mind. Problems of food storage, faulty diet, disease, and injury, as well as the adjustment of the mind necessary to live in constrained and crowded quarters for month after month, took their toll.

This book is about the devastation caused by these problems and about the people who tried to solve them.

I have not written this book just for the medical profession and have avoided medical terminology as much as possible. It is an account of seafaring history and the effort to sustain health aboard ships at sea, in the period of sailing ships on long voyages, up to the time of steam.

The barber-surgeons, apprenticed doctors, and medical graduates who diagnosed and treated diseases at sea were trained in the same schools as those practicing on land, and with similar doctrines and theories; they did so, however, under special circumstances: an inability to sequester the sick, close confinement, spoiled food, a limited diet, the ever-present stench of the bilge, and far greater deprivations than those known on land. Hardships included long exposure to the elements in torrid or frigid zones, as well as hostile natives and dietary inadequacies.

In the earliest years of this period, disease was understood to be inflicted on mankind by a wrathful God as punishment for humanity's transgressions, and cure was by means of prayer. Later, it was thought to be a contamination of the environment—the inhalation of vapors of putrefaction, mists arising from swamps and tidal flats, the sweat and body odors of people in cramped, poorly ventilated spaces. Any smell that was offensive signaled disease.

Later on, disease was thought to be the result of close association with sick people and an airborne toxic substance—often true enough, as far as it went—but the treatment was to remove the foreign material by bleeding, emetics, purgatives, and drugs that were thought to be antidotes. Against a few diseases, specifically effective medication had been identified: They knew about quinine for malaria, inoculation or vaccination for smallpox, mercurials for venereal problems.

A sailing ship on a long voyage offered its crew every opportunity for sickness except fresh contagion, and every port of call supplied that. Many vessels had no doctors, or only poorly trained ones who were unable to provide timely treatment even of the kind considered acceptable in the period. Against a backdrop of rampant epidemics, widespread disease, and brutal naval warfare between the sixteenth and the early part of the nineteenth centuries, naval medicine coped with terrible conditions, with little knowledge to support it. Even in this *enlightened* period, in which Newton and Harvey flourished, doctors had no understanding of disease or its effective treatment. As with wound healing, they knew only that some measures appeared to help and others did not. How sea surgeons coped this way for nearly three hundred years is both shocking and inspiring.

I am in debt to the many libraries that provided services to me. They include the library of the College of Physicians of Philadelphia, the Library Company of Philadelphia, and the library of the American Philosophical Society and the Independence Seaport Museum. In Britain, the services of the Wellcome Library and the library of the National Maritime Museum at Greenwich, as well as the library of the British Museum, were courteously offered. I received assistance from many sources but particularly wish to thank Charles Greifenstein and Chris Stanwood of the College of Physicians and Michael Angelo of the Independence Seaport Museum. Lastly, my wife Kathie gave inestimable help in reviewing the text.

Medicine Under Sail

Chapter 1

The Origins of Naval Medicine

I N THE Trojan wars, when Menelaus was wounded by a Trojan bowman, his brother and fleet commander Agamemnon sent for his fleet surgeon, Machaon, the son of Aesculapius, the god of medicine, to treat the wound. His treatment was described by Homer in the *Iliad*, book 4:

> Without delay he drew
> the arrow from the fairly fitted belt.
> The barbs were bent in drawing.
> Then he loosed the plate—the armorer's work—and carefully
> O'er looked the wound where fell the bitter shaft,
> Cleansed it from blood, and sprinkled over it
> with skill the soothing balsam of yore which
> the friendly Chiron to his father gave.

Before the modern era, there was a long tradition of naval surgeons who were called upon to treat the injured and the sick. In the early days of western civilization, the navies of Greece, Rome, and the Italian city-states assigned medical men to their ships of war. During the period of the Roman Empire, practitioners of medicine and surgery were assigned to each trireme, one for each two hundred men.

In the reign of the Emperor Hadrian (A.D. 117–38), there was an acute shortage of medical practitioners, and it was necessary to double their pay to attract them to the navy. In the fleets based at Ravenna and Miscerium, the term *duplicarius* followed the name of the medical attendant. Originally, their pay was 450 denari a month, but it was gradually increased to a thousand denari.

By the eleventh century, barber-surgeons had taken over the task of surgery in Mediterranean navies and were known in Italy as barbaries, and their assistants, barbarietos. Barbariers accompanied ships trading with England, and the practice of appointing barber-surgeons to ships spread to English ships.[1]

In England, before the reign of Henry VIII, there was no national navy. If a dispute with a foreign power required a naval force, merchant ships were impressed and soldiers boarded to fight the enemy.

The Venetian and Genoese galleys and carracks that frequently visited England and Flanders inspired Henry VIII to build his own navy. He employed Italian shipwrights to work in English yards. Once built, the ships were captained by the nobility under an agreement of indenture. The surgeons in this fleet were barber-surgeons and regarded as common sailors until they were given a warrant in 1704. Warrants were also issued to others requiring technical training, such as pilots, boatswains, carpenters, and gunners.

When Henry VIII ascended the throne, the practice of medicine and surgery was chaotic. Those involved as healers included physicians, surgeons, and barber-surgeons, in addition to pharmacists and itinerant quacks. Physicians were associated with universities and the Catholic Church, but the latter relation ended under Henry's edicts. The physicians regarded surgeons and pharmacists as inferior, lacking classical education, but the surgeons and the barber-surgeons provided such necessary services that they continued to thrive. They became so skillful in removing stones from the bladder and kidneys, setting fractures, and treating wounds that monarchs depended on them to treat seamen and soldiers wounded in battle.

To bring order to this chaos, the king granted collegiate rights and the power to grant licenses to physicians, surgeons, and apothecaries, who were to organize all others in the healing arts. Physicians were university graduates; surgeons at this time had served as an apprentice to a surgeon; apothecaries also had served an apprenticeship. The barber-surgeons were amalgamated into the Company of Barber-Surgeons in 1540 and kept under the supervision of the physicians; the apothecaries were organized into the City Company of Spices, likewise controlled by the physicians.

The barber-surgeons, because of their services to the crown in times of war, received special dispensation; they need not carry arms and were exempted from inquests and from town watch but could be pressed into service. The graduates of the Company of Barber-Surgeons who practiced surgery were under the supervision of the Royal College of Physicians

(1518) but were not permitted to practice bleeding, although they had much experience in treating injuries, wounds, and fractures.[2] The primary interest of the College of Physicians, with respect to the barber-surgeons, was to limit their activities so that they did not compete with the physicians.

Developing the Profession

The Spanish were in advance of the English in recognizing the importance of physicians. In the Spanish Armada there were eighty-five physicians and surgeons, as well as hospital ships.[3]

Prior to Elizabeth I, who reigned from 1558 to 1603, no physician served on any British ship; only barber-surgeons were aboard. One of them, William Clowes, published a book in 1596, *A Profitable and Necessary Booke of Observation for all those that are Burned with the Flame of Gunpowder and also for the Curing of Wounds made with Musket and Cavaliere Shot.* This was the first English text on military and naval surgery. In the book, Clowes complained of surgeons' lack of training and stated, "There is no coine so current but hath in it some counterfeits, which makes it suspicious; so there is no profession so good, but hath also some counterfeits which breed in it, disgrace . . . and some that take upon them the honest title and names of travelling surgeons, . . . nay these are idle and ignorant menslaiers."

Clowes also showed the folly of having a surgeon on board without medical training. The Royal College prohibited barber-surgeons from practicing medicine. Yet, when at sea, the surgeon was responsible for the sick as well as the injured. Clowes treated the daughter of the "Emperor," who was on her way to marry King Philip of Spain when she sustained a fractured rib with pleuritic pain, in the stormy weather on the "narrow sea." He complained, "There was not at that time any physitian in the navy to aid and assist me in this cure."[4]

Barber-surgeons became more secure in their position during the reign of Charles I, who reigned from 1625 to 1649. Charles gave Thomas Woodall (see chapter 2) the responsibility for providing barber-surgeons to all of his ships. In addition to their surgical skills, barber-surgeons still trimmed beards and cut hair. Woodall stated, "There belongeth to the Surgeon's Mate a carefull and especial respect to be had concerning scissors; namely, that he have at least two paires of good scissors for to cut hair. . . . as also in his box, one paire for use in surgery . . . for the Surgeon's Mate by due consignment is to be the Barber of the Ships Company."[5]

In this early period, John Moyle, a surgeon in the Royal Navy, wrote about the duties of the surgeon in preparation for battle:

> I will imagine that you are now at sea in a Man-of-War and in sight of the enemy and all men are clearing their respective quarters . . . at what time as you are chyrurgeon of the ship, you must prepare as followeth. First, seeth your Allop or Platform be laid as even as possible with a sail spread smooth upon it, which you must speak to the Commander to order. In Merchantmen the chyrurgeon's place is usually in the Cable Tier between decks, but in Men-of-War in the Hold abaft of the mast between that and the Bulkhead of the Cockpit, from side to side. In this place, you must have two chests to set your wounded on to dress them, and at the corner of the platform you are to place two vessels, one with water to wash hands between each operation and to wet your dismembering bladders in and for other services, and the other to throw amputated limbs until you have the opportunity to heave them overboard.
>
> You must likewise place good store of lights above your platform on Lanthorns, by two of the largest in the place you are to operate.
>
> There must be in readiness instruments, astringent powders, rowlers [roller bandages] bolsters, tow, acetum, broad tape, ligatures, and splints.
>
> Also basons to mix your restrictives in, pannikins to warm your oyles in . . . cordial bittles ready at hand to relieve men when they fraint.

Captain John Smith (1580–1631), of Virginia and Pocahontas fame, mentioned the duties of a surgeon and the surviving crew after a naval battle:

> Chirurgeon, look to the wounded, and winde up the slain, with each a bullet or weight at their heads and feet to make them sink, and give them three gunnes for their funeral. Swabbers, make cleane the ship. Pursers record their names. Gunners, sponge your ordinance. Soldiers, scour leakes; Boatswain and the rest, repair sails and shrouds; Cooke see you observe the morning watch; Boy, fetch my cellar of bottles. Master, lay him safe in board laufe for laufe; Midshipmen, see the tops and yards well manned. [6]

Professional Status

Until 1745 the Company of Barber-Surgeons continued to examine and appoint surgeons to the Royal Navy. This system finally became untenable because the surgeons' training was confined to the treatment of casualties, without knowledge of the treatment of disease. When the captain of a ship complained to his surgeon about the high mortality from disease, his complaint was forwarded to the Company of Barber-Surgeons, who replied they had no knowledge of disease and could take no responsibility. The College of Physicians, in protecting their own interests, had refused to allow barber-surgeons to treat disease—except when at sea, as the physicians had no inclination to live on board and provide medical care.

The precipitating incident that led Parliament to order the navy to discontinue appointing barber-surgeons and to request the College of Surgeons to provide future naval surgeons who were also trained in medicine was the imprisonment of a barber-surgeon, Neil Stewart, by the French when his ship was captured. Stewart requested transfer from the seamen's prison to the officers' prison and showed his warrant. After the passage of several days without any action being taken, he again spoke to his translator and was told that the prison superintendent did not know whether he was a barber or a surgeon. The French navy had long since discontinued the use of barber-surgeons. The case of Neil Stewart was regarded as an affront to the nation.[7]

In 1745 those doctors trained as surgeons, having been apprenticed to a physician and surgeon, or having a medical degree and having practiced surgery, separated from the barber-surgeons and formed their own guild known as the Company of Surgeons. In addition to not practicing as barbers, they had taken courses in anatomy, botany, and chemistry as well as surgery. The new Company of Surgeons now examined candidates for the navy.

By 1780 most candidates who took the navy qualifying examination were graduates from a medical school with a baccalaureate in medicine or a medical degree. Most were from the Scottish medical schools of Edinburgh, Glasgow, or Aberdeen, prompting Samuel Johnson's remark, "Much may be made of a Scotsman if he be caught young."[8]

To get a medical degree from Oxford or Cambridge, a student first had to complete seven years of courses in Greek, Latin, and Hebrew and receive a master of arts degree, before enrolling in a medical school that taught the ancient philosophical medicine of Galen and Paracelsus. The Scottish schools taught clinical medicine and required hospital rotations.

Peter Cullen described, in the third person, his examination for the post of a naval surgeon by the Company of Surgeons in 1789.

[T]he examiners were seated at a semi circular table. . . . Mr. Cullen having walked up to the table and made his bow was asked his name, from whence he came, for what purpose. . . . On answering it was for the naval service, one of the examiners rose and taking Mr. Cullen to the side of the room, enquired his age, his apprenticeship, studies, and practice in the profession . . . the examiner proceeded to question him in anatomy, physiology, and surgery . . . and asked how he would treat certain surgical cases. . . . This gentleman was quite satisfied . . . and taking him to the centre of the table where the president was sitting said, "I find this young gentleman fully qualified as an Assistant Surgeon for His Majesty's Navy." The president bowed to Mr. Cullen and desired him to pay one guinea as a fee, and asked him to call the next day at the Navy Office where he would find his certificate.[9]

The Company of Surgeons was granted a royal charter in 1800 and thereafter was known as the Royal College of Surgeons. In the navy, at this time, the term *surgeon* was applied to all those engaged in the practice of medicine and surgery. When a surgeon was promoted to the position of chief medical officer of a fleet or a hospital, he was given the more exalted title of *physician*. It was not until 1805 that the Royal Navy authorized a uniform for medical officers, although they still received their warrants from the Navy Board, not the Admiralty, which only commissioned executive officers.[10]

Conflicts of Command: The Captain and the Surgeon

During most of the eighteenth century, the relationship between the captain and his senior officers with the ship's surgeon was often one-sided, with the captain making decisions affecting health without asking any advice from the surgeon. In the early 1700s, the surgeon had little to contribute toward the effective control of disease, and the indifference of the captain and his officers to his suggestions had little effect on the outcome either way. However, later, when enough information was known so that the spread of disease could be limited by the recommendations of the surgeon, captains who failed to heed their suggestions paid a price; they met the enemy with a crew unduly debilitated and dispirited with sickness.

The surgeon held a warrant, was not even a commissioned officer, and rarely succeeded in having his protests reach the captain. If the surgeon noted the outbreak of cases of scurvy and requested a stopover on an island to gather fresh food supplies, or if the anchorage was in an unhealthy part of the harbor and a change of anchorage indicated, he could be overruled by the captain. He could recommend against the transfer of men from a diseased ship or accepting impressed replacements, but his requests were usually ignored until too late.

It was customary for many commissioned officers to manifest a strict and distant behavior toward medical officers. Some of this prejudice was related to the lowly origins of the early surgeons and their barber-surgeon past. Ship's officers also often looked down upon surgical practice as a manual occupation equated with carpenters, sail-makers, or gunners. Also, while there were many well-trained and brilliant naval surgeons, there were also surgeons whose lack of training and character made them unqualified to support a medical practice and who sought refuge in the navy. Some, having apprenticed with an apothecary, passed the examinations at the Royal College of Surgeons, although they might be ignorant of anatomy or surgery. Often a lack of the proper background made it impossible to acquire the manners of a gentleman, and surgeons on board were sometimes regarded by officers of the quarterdeck as inferior.

The ability of the surgeon to prevent, control, and treat shipboard diseases had so improved near the close of the eighteenth century, as had the realization that health was an important factor in determining victory or defeat, that the surgeon, at last, was regarded as a key player in naval warfare. The control of disease on shipboard at this time was a medical revolution. Yet he was still powerless to act unless the commanding officer recognized his skills and importance. Unfortunately, many fleet commanders and captains held the surgeon in such low esteem that he continued to be ignored. If his suggestions disturbed the daily schedule or broke with tradition, they fell on deaf ears. Yet, the most brilliant and successful naval engagements were won by commanders who heeded the advice of their surgeons.

At the Battle of the Saints in the Caribbean, Gilbert Blane, fleet surgeon (see chapter 2), and Admiral Rodney worked closely together, and with a healthy crew scored a decisive victory over the diseased French fleet under the command of Admiral DeGrasse. Blane, like Trotter (see chapter 2), was a personal physician to the fleet commander, and it was by this means that he achieved his status. The only illness among the British seamen occurred when they manned the disease-ridden French prizes. The British battle casualties were 266 killed and 810 injured, of whom 88 subsequently died of tetanus (lockjaw). Although tetanus, a common complication of a gunshot wound, must have been seen often in battle casualties, it is rarely mentioned in this period.

Blane had been given full freedom of the quarterdeck and often discussed health matters with the senior officers. He described having breakfast on the deck with Rodney and captains Sir Charles Douglas, Simmons, and Lord Cranston on the morning of the battle. The latter remarked that if the wind held, they could pass through the enemy's line of ships. Rodney heard this remark but made no comment. When the battle began, he implemented this tactic; it was the first time it was employed.

After the battle, Douglas introduced Blane to DeGrasse as the doctor who was *assez habile pour faire revivre les morts* [who could revive the dead]. DeGrasse, as might be anticipated, had little regard for doctors and replied, "*Et peutêtre pour faire mourir les vivants*" [and perhaps to kill the living].[11]

As a warrant officer, a surgeon was classed as a civilian craftsman like the purser or chaplain. Not being commissioned, he was often denied the quarterdeck, which was reserved for commissioned officers. In 1805, when a uniform was prescribed for surgeons in the British navy, he became a gentlemen, but it was not until 1843 that he was granted a commission. Uniforms for seamen were not prescribed in the Royal Navy until 1857, but long before that, as far back as the Tudor period, seamen could be recognized by their dress, and some captains prescribed and paid for uniforms for their crews. The captain of HMS *Blazer* had his men wear blue and white striped jerseys, and thus the term *blazer*.[12]

Surgeons' Compensation

In the British and American navies in the 1700s, the surgeon not only was responsible for medical treatment of the crew but also had to provide medicines and procure instruments, paying for these out of his own pocket. A conscientious surgeon administering treatment on a sickly ship could thus end the year in debt. To offset his medical expenses, the surgeon in the Royal Navy received five shillings monthly, and each crewmember had two pence per month subtracted from his pay to be collected by the surgeon.

In the reign of Queen Anne, a bounty or free gift was granted to each surgeon to help defray the cost of medication. Queen Anne's bounty continued long after her death and was increased in time of war, the amount depending on the size of the ship. In 1770, the bounty to the surgeon for a third-rate ship, with a crew of six hundred men, was forty-three shillings a year. Marines assigned to a ship and army units being transported did not pay into the medical fund to the surgeon, but he was still responsible for their medical treatment. Robertson, surgeon on the *Edgar* during an

eighteen-month assignment in peacetime, spent 148 shillings on medicines while his pay and perquisites totaled 302 shillings.[13]

Five hundred British surgeons cared for the health of the fleet and treated diseases and wounds during the Napoleonic wars, but with the imprisonment of Napoleon on Elba, three hundred were summarily discharged
to reduce expenses. These doctors were turned loose without jobs or compensation. It was recommended to the Sick and Wounded Board that
shore medical installations used by the Royal Navy provide work for these
discharged doctors. Surgeons with five or more years of service were to
provide treatment in naval hospitals, dockyards, and prison ships. Robertson, Trotter, and others urged the board to pay a pension to discharged
surgeons of about three shillings sixpence daily, based on their service.
They would remain in the reserve and forfeit their pensions when called
back to active duty.

The Admiralty received many such proposals before the king and council finally acted in April 1805. The new regulations paid surgeons in active
service six shillings sixpence daily in home waters and increased the payment to seven shillings sixpence for those in foreign stations, with increases based on length of service. Widows of surgeons who were killed or
who died in service were to receive sixteen pounds annually. Pensions
were based upon length of service and after twenty years topped at six
shillings a day.

Chapter 2

Practicing Medicine at Sea

NAVAL MEDICINE in the age of sail comes down to us in quaint language that expresses many attitudes and assumptions that we know to be false. Even so, the courage and intelligence of the sea surgeons shine clear. Between the gore and agony of battle and the dignified indifference of the Admiralty, they searched for the truth of disease and healing, often coming very close to the mark.

Thomas Woodall (1569–1643)

The teachings of brilliant men are often lost in the dusty archives of time, only to be rediscovered generations later at great cost to humanity. Sometimes the neglect is due to the lack of publication of their ideas, or failure to promote them sufficiently. At other times, truth was submerged by strident soothsayers, faddist doctrines, or an audience unwilling to be disturbed by a new idea. Sometimes truth was buried because it was planted on unprepared, infertile soil and so failed to flower in an age of little interest. Thomas Woodall's insights arose in such an age.

Thomas Woodall deserves the title of "Father of Marine Medicine," not only for his on-target observations on scurvy, the dreaded disease of seamen, but for his advanced views on wounds, fractures, and amputations. His prescient views matured from his experiences as a traveler on the European continent, where he was known for his treatment of plague victims, from his many arduous trips as a ship surgeon to the East Indies, and from his teaching commitments and books for young students. Charles I of England, in recognition of his achievements, thrust on him the responsibilities of organizing medical support for the British fleet. In response, Woodall laid the foundations for naval medicine and was among the first to recommend the juice of citrus fruits as a preventive and cure for scurvy.

Woodall as Teacher

Woodall stated his advanced ideas in several books, including *A Treatise on Gangrene and Sphacelos, Viaticum,* and *A Treatise on the Plague,* all published in 1653, after his death. He also wrote *The Surgeon's Mate,* which was a textbook for students that discussed marine medicine and surgery. As a prominent surgeon, he was a leader in the Company of Barber-Surgeons, in which position he succeeded in having Charles I grant the group a new royal charter. When selected by the king to be a medical consultant to the Royal Navy, he immediately recommended and received an increased pay scale for surgeons.

In this office, Woodall also promulgated a code of conduct for barber-surgeons on joining the navy. The first duty of the surgeon was to God; second, he must respect his superiors, supporting them with diligent, careful efforts, not exposing their weaknesses, keeping their remedies secret, and remaining faithful to their orders; third, he had to be skilled in his calling, to read and be learned in "physick and chirurgy." Referring his students to their first duty, he stated: "There are . . . the three great arrowes of the Almighty . . . to cut sinners from the Earth in all ages and in all nations. . . . The three arrowes are War, Famine, and Pestilence."[1]

Woodall had studied the works of Galen, Mesues, Avicenna, Tegaltus, Vigo, and Paracelsus. However, his teachings departed from the path of these oracles and were the result of a long period of practical experience, careful observations, and considered judgment. Woodall divided all wounds into three categories. The first category was puncture wounds from the thrust of a dagger or rapier; he had no classification for a lacerated wound and must have included it in puncture wounds. His second type of wound was a gunshot wound, and the third was that associated with a fracture of a bone. The first dressing of a wound was "to remove unnatural things forced into the wound . . . which should be done with the least pain to the patient and avoiding arteries, nerves, and veins." These unnatural things would include wood splinters from the spars and masts, as well as metal fragments from cannon fire. If removal was deemed difficult or caused too much pain—there was no anesthesia—he recommended that his students "tarry if you may, while nature helps."

Woodall instructed that balm was to be applied to the wound, and if bleeding was excessive, an attempt should be made to ligate the bleeding vessel. Dressings soaked in wine were then placed over the wound. (The alcohol in wine could act as an antiseptic.) If fever developed, and it usually did, bleeding and purging were recommended. The new treatment of wounds advanced by Ambroise Paré, the great French military surgeon, was taught by Woodall. Paré's and Woodall's treatment was a departure from the usual treatment of wounds, which was by cauterization with hot oil and the searing iron.

When the patient is overcome by a wound infection, he wrote, the fever would rise and the pain would become worse when pus was in the making, but once the infection subsided, the patient had less pain and the fever declined as pressure in the tissues diminished.

In Woodall's time gunpowder, first used in battle in the fourteenth century, was thought to be poisonous; such wounds went on to "corruption" and gangrene. He taught that, if gangrene were to develop in a limb, "there will be an extinction of the lively colour . . . grievous pain . . . and sometimes putrid discharge, and on being opened a filthy ichor of an unsavoury smell proceeding from it." This required medicines and bleeding to offset the poisons, but with such wounds he also adamantly refrained from the usual treatment of boiling oil.

Woodall was not of a mind to amputate limbs with gunshot wounds forthwith, either, which was the custom of many surgeons in that period and for several hundred years afterward. He taught that amputation is to be reserved only for those cases where more than one-half the limb was dismembered, or in the presence of a chronic discharging, suppurating wound, or if the patient's life was endangered or the remaining parts of the limb were not serviceable. His concepts were far more conservative and reasonable than those of military surgeons two hundred years later during the Civil War in America, who favored immediate amputation of any limb with a gunshot wound. "For it is no small presumption to dismember the image of God." But, when an amputation is needed and the surgery done, the patient is improved ". . . as a tree is made better when the dead boughs are pruned."

Woodall recommended an amputation four inches below the knee even if only the foot is "corrupted." The stump is better and the pain the same, regardless of the level, but the level must be at least four inches above the gangrenous part. A surgical student today would be exposed to similar teaching.

In India Woodall had observed judicial amputations of the leg and foot as punishment for crimes, after which the criminal could walk with a prosthesis of reeds filled with cotton; he prescribed such prostheses for his patients. He pointedly commented that great personages rarely do as well after an amputation as do the weak, indigent, and miserable.

Woodall defined an intermediate state of health between life and death—a state of disability when the bloom of health has faded. "For from the beginning, all men are constituted to dye, and yet there is an interim for each man of not being in health, neither really dead but, '*quasi moriens*' . . . dying or half dying."

Discussing fractures of bones he wrote, "The first intention is the cure of a fracture, and is performed by restoring the bone disjoyned." The second intention was to keep the divided ends together until healed. The third intention was the curing of the wound. The fourth intention is "to prevent or remove the accident." Did this fourth intention mean an analysis of the cause of the accident and measures to be taken to prevent its recurrence? If so, Woodall was opening a new frontier in the medicine of his century; he was entering the area of public health and preventive medicine, an aspect of medical practice alien to this period and the following century.

Woodall was an avowed teacher. In all of his writings, student instructions appeared to be his primary purpose, and he repeatedly addressed students in his texts. The novice was taught the intricacies of medicine, and he guided students in the planning of a surgical procedure, promulgating six cardinal rules. First, before acting, get a consultation; two, do not delay surgery; three, always act with permission of the patient, and if the patient can't reason responsibly, get a consent from his friends or kindred; four, have experience with the operation; five, all equipment must be ready; six, before beginning an operation, the surgeon and his assistants were to call upon God for a blessing. His teachings emphasized careful observation, deliberation to avoid precipitous decisions, careful wound treatment, respect for the patient, and attention to details.

Woodall Practicing Medicine

Much of Woodall's instruction bore directly on the handling of accidents and battle wounds aboard ship. He wrote from extensive experience.

When a sailor fell from a mast or spar to the deck, Woodall warned, the surgeon was frequently presented with a skull fracture or brain injury. The injured seaman could present "with lethargie or frenzie, madnesse, losse of memory, deadish sleep, giddinesse, apoplexie, paralysis and divers other like accidents." Such a description of the various states of consciousness can only come from a person well experienced in seeing such injuries. Treatment of such an injury remained unchanged in the seventeenth and through the nineteenth centuries: desiccation and cicatrization of the wound with local medications. If the bones of the skull were collapsed on the brain, the surgeon elevated the depressed fragments and removed the bone splinters. Wounds of the chest and abdomen were beyond the surgeon's ministrations, and in the hands of God.

If the victim fell into the sea or was washed overboard and was fortunate enough to be hauled back on deck, he would be held upside down by his heels and shaken to remove the water from his chest.

A hundred years later, James Lind (see chapter four) had better success. He wrapped the victim in a blanket and rolled him about the deck; the extremities were massaged, the patient was bled, and warm air was blown into the lungs by bellows (or, sometimes, the breath of a person chewing garlic was the source of the air). The nostrils of the victim were pinched closed, while a second person alternatively pressed on the ribs to mimic breathing.[2] This treatment was later recommended by the Humane Societies in both England and America. Humane Societies also proposed this treatment for those struck by lightning or those rendered unconscious by inhaling toxic vapors used in the disinfection of ships. Such vapors might be burning gunpowder, pitch, or vinegar fumes.

Woodall taught that the primary cause of disease was sin, followed by venomous, toxic, and stinking vapors from stagnant bilge water. Slaughterhouses and putrid objects were also regarded as causing disease. Such concepts were common to most physicians in this period and for the next 150 years were thought to be the origin of most diseases. To remain healthy, one should (besides living a moral life) avoid foul-smelling vapors, give cemeteries a wide berth, and guard against the night air.

Woodall suggested hot bayberries carried on a hot shovel and deposited in each room to purify the air. Along with other physicians, he prescribed a perforated box within which there was a sponge soaked in wine, vinegar, rosemary, lemon, and cloves. Once disease was contracted, a solution of sage, pepper, ginger, and nutmeg was to be taken twice daily. Foul odors caused disease and aromatic ones cured it.

Regarded as an expert in the treatment of plague, having been involved in such an epidemic during his travels in Poland, Woodall discussed plague as vengeance from God.

> Such is God's miraculous hand in his various and unsearchable ways of affecting Mankind in that most noisome disease of the Pestilence, that it is not only wonderful, but impossible for the wit of many, however wise or learned he may esteem himself or by others be esteemed, to give a sufficient reason, with also a methodical cure for that most contagious noisome and killing disease of the Pestilence. . . . Yet He has given us leave and judgment to take lawful means to preserve our frail bodies. . . . *Flagellum Dei pro peccates Mundi.*

If, for Woodall, the plague was the rod of God for the sins of the world, he had the full support of the Church. The clergy also preached that plague and other diseases represented the wrath of God levied on sinful mankind; the suffering must be borne. But Woodall, like other physicians in all ages, did not believe that people should bow their heads and passively accept the consequences of God's wrath but should use God-given knowledge to overcome the curse. The privy council of the city of Westminster gave Woodall a medal for a pill he prescribed, which was said to have saved sixty people afflicted by the plague in 1638.[3]

Sailing with the Explorers

Whenever large numbers of people were crowded together, diseases appeared, and this problem was recognized in the earliest assemblage of a crew on a vessel in the fifteenth century. It continued to be a major determinant in victory or defeat at sea, as well as the success or failure of the voyages of exploration, which shaped the destiny of nations during this period of colonial expansion. Improving conditions on board had practical value, all altruistic considerations aside, but the authorities were slow to recognize it.

In the earliest days of Queen Elizabeth I's navy, problems due to sickness plagued the Admiralty. Lord Charles Howard in 1588 wrote to Lord Burghley about the overwhelming incidence of sickness and the lack of care for crew members, describing how ill crewmembers were abandoned in the streets of Margate and left to die. Howard went ashore and tried to ameliorate their sufferings, using his own funds to arrange for shelter in barns or outhouses. "It would grieve any man's heart to see them that have served so valiantly to die so miserably."

In the same period, Sir Walter Raleigh (1554–1618) remarked that seamen went with a "great grudging to serve his Majesty's ships as if it were to be slaves in a galley."[4]

Forty-one years after Howard's complaint, in 1629, another captain, Sir Henry Mervin, writing to the Lords Commissioners of the Admiralty, pleaded for better conditions for oceangoing crews: "I beseech your Lordships . . . take speedy course for the redress . . . for foul winter months, naked backs and empty bellies make the common man voice the King's service [James I] worse than galley slavery. . . ." Mervin echoes Raleigh in warning, "Let not your eyes that look on the common public good, overlook this mischief, for without better order, his Majesty will lose the love and loyalty of his sailors and the Royal Navy will droop. I beseech your Lordships, pardon plainness that proceeds from an honest heart; for the disease admits no palliative physic."[5]

Sir Francis Drake (1540?–1596)

The elaborate expeditions of Francis Drake and John Hawkins against the Spanish settlements in the West Indies failed because of a sudden contagion that killed so many men that the military objectives had to be curtailed. Drake wrote in his journal:

> From hence putting over to the West Indies, we were not many dayes at Sea but there began amongst our people such mortality, as in a few dayes there were dead above two or three hundred men. And until some, seven or eight dayes after our coming from Saint Jago, there had not dyed any one man of sicknesse in all the Fleet: the sicknesse shewed not his infection, wherewith so many were stroken untill we were departed thence, and there seazed our people with extreme hot burning and continuall ague, whereof some very few escaped with life and yet those for the most part not without great alteration and decay of their wits and strength for a long time after. In some that dyed were plainly shewn the small spots, which are often found upon those that be infective with Plague.

From Drake's description, a specific diagnosis is not possible, but typhus, cholera, yellow fever, and bubonic plague must be considered.[6] They stopped for six weeks while more of his company died and the survivors remained weak, "decayed in their memory," and convinced that the night air at St. Jago had infected them with this "very burning and pestilent Ague." The "inconvenience of continuall mortality" forced the expedition to turn home without "full recompence of our tedious travailes." [7]

Drake carried a surgeon on his expeditions to the West Indies. However, after the surgeon died they seemed to have managed the deadly consequences of an ambush rather well on their own, giving due credit to divine intervention:

> The generall himself was shot in the face under his right eye and close by his nose, the arrow piercing a marvellous way in under *basis cerebri* with no small danger of his life besides that, he was grievously wounded in the head. The rest being nine persons in the boat, were deadly wounded in divers parts of their bodies, if God almost miraculously had not give cure to the same. For our chief Surgeon being dead and the others absent by the loss of our vice-admirall, and having none left us but a boy, whose good will was more than any skil he had, we were little better than altogether destitute of such cunning and helps as so grievous a state of so many wounded bodies did require. Notwith standing God, by the very good advice of our Generall and the diligent putting too of every man's help, did give such speedy and wonderful cures, that we had all great comfort thereby and yeilded God the glory, whereof.[8]

Surgeons in Battle

Baron von Swieten, an Austrian military surgeon, discussed treatment of war wounds in his textbook, *The Diseases Incident to Armies*. Excerpts from this book regarding naval warfare were published by William Northcote in America in 1776 and entitled *Extracts from the Marine Practice of Physic and Surgery for the Military and Naval Surgeons*. His instructions reflect an only slightly advanced state of the art, more than a hundred years after John Moyle and John Smith (see chapter 1) offered their advice.

It advised naval surgeons to have in a state of readiness a chest that contained tourniquets and needles of all sizes, including crooked needles, as well as a large quantity of lint (some of it mixed with flour to absorb drainage), double and single roller bandages, thread, "pledgets [compresses] of taw [tow, linen fibers]," splints and bolsters, and tape to secure them.

In sighting an enemy ship, the surgeon was to ask the captain for part of the ship to use as a surgical operating and dressing station. The carpenter laid a platform covered with a stretched sail; seamen's bedding was placed on the platform. This area was usually the cockpit, a part of the lowest deck just above the hold. Some beds were also collected, in case officers were wounded. The surgeon was to now assemble his mates and assistants to consult on treatment. He might ask for additional personnel from the first mate for help in transporting the injured.

As the cannonading began, if several wounded arrived simultaneously, triaging was accomplished by treating the most serious cases first; otherwise the surgical team was to dress the wounded as they arrived, without distinction. Northcote relayed the Baron's advice: "You should use expedition, but don't hurry. In respect to the wounded you should act as if you were entirely unaffected by their groans and complaints, but behave with caution, not rashly or cruelly, nor cause any unnecessary pain. Never encourage those with slight wounds to remain out of action, but insist they return to their stations; otherwise threaten to report them to their officers after the engagement."

It was also the duty of the surgeon to dispose of the dead. The slain, weighted with cannon shot tied to them, one to the head and one to the feet to make them sink, are thrown overboard at the end of the battle after their names are recorded by the purser, just as Captain John Smith described in the early seventeenth century. Three guns were fired as a tribute, as the bodies sank. The names of the casualties were recorded in the surgeon's journal, which was used as a reference later in determining compensation claims.

After the battle, the surgeon reported to the captain the number and prognosis of the casualties, and the seriously wounded would be transferred to shore hospitals when such were available.[9]

Surgeons' Journals and Reports

The few extant journals of surgeons that recount their experiences during battle provide a good insight into the problems they experienced.

Edward Ives

Surgeon Edward Ives on Admiral Watson's flagship described the turmoil in the cockpit during a battle fought in the Indian Ocean in 1755.

At the very instant I was amputating the limb of one wounded seaman, I met with an almost continuous interruption from the rest of his companions, who were in the like distressed circumstances, some pouring forth the most piercing cries to be taken care of, while others seized my arm in their earnestness of being relieved even at the time I was passing the needle for securing a divided blood vessel by a ligature. Surely at the time such operations are in contemplation, the operator's mind as well as body ought to be as little agitated as possible; and the very shaking of the lower gun deck owing to the recoil of the large cannon which are placed just over his head is of itself sufficient to incommode a surgeon.

Ives asked the captain to erect the platform lower in the ship, in the hold if necessary, where it would be quieter and safer for the surgeon and the wounded.[10]

Robert Young

In a journal that remained unpublished until 1961, Robert Young, surgeon of the *Ardent* during the Battle of Camperdown in 1797, vividly described his work in the cockpit. He had no mates to assist him.

All of these were wounded in the action of October 11, in which I had no mate, having been without one for three months before. I was employed in operating and dressing till near 4.0 in the morning, the action beginning about 1.0 in the afternoon. So great was my fatigue that I began several amputations under a dread of sinking before I should have secured the blood vessels.

Ninety wounded were brought down during the action. The whole cockpit deck, cabins, wing berths and part of the cable tier, together with my platform and my preparations for dressing were covered with them. So that for a time they were laid on each other at the foot of the ladder where they were brought down, and I was obliged to go on deck to the Commanding Officer to state the situation and apply for men to go down the main hatchway and move the foremost of the wounded further forward into the tiers and wings and thus make room in the cockpit. Numbers, about sixteen mortally wounded, died after they were brought down, amongst whom was the brave and worthy Captain Burgess, whose corpse could with difficulty be conveyed to the starboard wing berth.

Joseph Bonheur had his right thigh taken off by a cannon shot close to the pelvis, so that it was impossible to apply a tourniquet; his right arm was also shot to pieces. The stump of the thigh, which was very fleshy, presented a dreadful and large surface of mangled flesh. In this state he lived near two hours, perfectly sensible and incessantly called out in a strong voice to me to assist him. The bleeding from the femoral artery, although so high up, must have been very inconsiderable, and I observed it did not bleed as he lay. All the service I could render this unfortunate man was to put dressing over the part and give him drink.

In many other instances I had occasion to observe that vessels collapse and bleed little after gunshot or splinter wounds. The vessel probably stretched longitudinally has its sides brought more together, and the cavity diminished; when at length transversely separated by violence, the jagged ends detract inwards, which with the spasmodic contraction of the circular fibres of the artery, occasioned by the tension, completely closes the passage and resists the impetus of the blood from above. Whether this attempt to describe be just or not, the fact is deserving of notice.

Melancholy cries for assistance were addressed to me from every side by wounded and dying, and piteous moans and bewailing from pain and despair. In the midst of these agonising scenes, I was able to preserve myself firm and collected, and embracing in my mind the whole of the situation, to direct my attention where the greatest and most essential services could be performed. Some with wounds, bad indeed and painful, but slight in comparison with the dreadful condition of others, were most vociferous for my assistance. These I was obliged to reprimand with severity, as their voices disturbed the last moments of the dying. I cheered and commended the patient fortitude of others, and sometimes extorted a smile of satisfaction from the mangled sufferers, and succeeded to those momentary gleams of cheerfulness amidst so many horrors. The man whose leg I had first amputated had not uttered a groan from the time he was brought down, and several, exulting in the news of the victory, declared they regretted not the loss of their limbs.

An explosion of a salt box with several cartridges abreast of the cockpit hatchway filled the hatchway with flame and in a moment 14 or 15 wretches tumbled down upon each other, their faces black as a cinder, their clothes blown to shatters and their hats on fire. A Corporal of Marines lived two hours after the action with all the glutei muscle shot away, so as to excavate the pelvis. Captain Burgess' wound was of this nature, but he fortunately died almost instantly.

After the action ceased, 15 or 16 dead bodies were removed before it was possible to get a platform cleared and come to the materials for operating and dressing, those I had prepared being covered over with bodies and blood, and the store room door blocked up.

I have the satisfaction to say that of those who survived to undergo amputation or be dressed, all were found the next morning in the gunroom, where they were placed, in as comfortable a state as possible, and on the third day were conveyed on shore in good spirits, cheering the ship at going away, smoking their pipes and jesting as they sailed along, and answering the cheers of thousands of the populace who received them on Yarmouth key. . . .

A man who is at once Physician, Surgeon and Apothecary, upon whom in these characters, the health and lives of so great a number of valuable subjects of the State are often solely depending, ought to have every means and every instrument and every accommodation to favour and aid the exercise of his industry and skill. . . .

The surgeon has every necessary article for his practice, but no conveniences for applying them with facility to use: he has plenty of ropes and sails, but no blocks or pulleys. For his necessaries, lime juice and gratuitous stores, the storeroom usually allotted is far too small. For making up and keeping at hand a regular formula of extemporaneous medicines, for having everything he may want ready of access, his instruments, lint, needles, his lotions, dressings, pills etc. etc. he has no convenience whatever. If in every ship of war a large store-room was allotted to the surgeon and in it a well contrived Dispensatory fitted up on a plan such as the Board might choose to adopt, to become part of the establishment of this department, all of which might very well be done in small, and in such a room as could easily be spared, a counter, with drawers below, and guarded shelves for bottles etc., I am convinced it would be more to a surgeon in a large ship than any of his three or four mates. I beg leave with earnestness to solicit the attention of the Board to this circumstance, which I am sure is of very great importance.

The expense would be trivial.

Signed: Robt. Young[11]

Of a complement of 485 men on board the *Ardent,* 41 were killed and 107 injured—more than a 30 percent casualty rate, which must have exhausted Young. Soon after this battle, Young contracted typhus and was separated from the service.

Sir Gilbert Blane

Sir Gilbert Blane was personal physician to Admiral Rodney with the British naval forces stationed in the West Indies between March 1780 and April 1783. Blane kept accurate records, and in his report to the Admiralty described the types of wounds incurred by seamen during different phases and tactics of naval warfare.

When ships dueled at long distances, well-directed cannonballs shredded the sails, splintered or severed masts, and littered the deck with debris. Wood splinters flew about, and shards of metal from fittings were hurled onto and across the deck.

Gun crews suffered scorches from spilled gunpowder scattered on the deck around the gun carriage and ignited by a shower of sparks when the gun was fired. Excess powder around the touchhole of a cannon could flare and burn those nearby. Other accidents occurred when gunpowder, rammed down the muzzle of the cannon when burning material from the previous firing still smoldered inside the gun, would explode prematurely, causing severe burns. Sometimes the barrel itself exploded and fragments of metal ripped across the deck. Of course, aside from accidents, burns were common incidents of battle when explosions set ships ablaze. Blane recommended linseed oil dressings for burns.

As the battling ships approached each other, the tactics and injury patterns changed. In close quarters there were fewer injured but a higher proportionate mortality. When closer still, a ball from the enemy's cannon penetrated the hull, whereas the spent ball fired from a distance splintered the wood and bounced off. Marine sharpshooters in the rigging took their toll of seamen on the deck. In grappling range, boarding parties leaped across the gunwales.

Blane reported that one quarter of all seamen killed or injured were from scorches (burns) from accidental explosions of gunpowder and made recommendations to prevent this. He also recommended to the Admiralty that each crewmember going into battle carry on his person a length of rope or garter to use as a tourniquet. As surgeon, he always carried several for the officers on the quarterdeck.[12]

Tobias Smollett's Roderick Ransom

A vivid depiction of a surgeon's life appears in the eighteenth-century novel, *Roderick Ransom,* by Tobias Smollett. Smollett had been a naval surgical mate before writing his novel, and from it much can be learned about the care of the sick aboard a warship. He wrote tellingly of the captain's view of the crew: "When he appeared on deck, the captain bade the doctor who stood bowing at his right hand, 'Look at these lazy lubberly son's of bitches who are good for nothing on board, but to eat the King's provisions and encourage idleness in skulkers.'"[13]

In this picaresque novel, Roderick Ransom, like Fielding's Tom Jones, roams the English countryside experiencing adventures that raise his hopes and misadventures that dash them, but the events of his medical career in the navy are too detailed not to have been experienced by Smollett himself. After an apprenticeship to a surgeon named Launcelot Crab, Ransom decides to join the navy as a surgeon's mate.

His examination is at Surgeons' Hall in London. Before he can take the examination, he learns he must pay tribute in bribes to the doorkeeper, the cleaning lady, the examiners, and the secretary.

The examiners asks Roderick, "What would you do to an injured arm?"

Ransom replies, "Bleed it." The examiners then huddle together and confer. They ask, "Would you not bind the arm, first?" Ransom agrees and passes the examination, but then is told that there were no openings in the navy. To get a position, he must pay additional bribe money.

Destitute and walking the streets of London, he is assaulted by a press gang, and when he recovers consciousness he is lying on the deck of HMS *Thunderer*. He befriends the chief surgeon's mate and is assigned to the cockpit as one of his assistants.

Shortly after, the surgeon's mates are drinking in the cockpit, and Morgan, a Welshman, the senior mate, is approached by a sailor who brings him a mate's prescription for filling. After a few more drinks, Morgan gets up and asks the sailor if his messmate was alive or dead, saying, "Jack, if he was dead, he would have no occasion for doctor stuff."

"No, thank God, death hasn't as yet boarded him, but they have been yardarm and yardarm these three glasses," the sailor replied. "His starboard eye is open, but fast jammed in his head; and the halyards of his lower jaw have given way."

When asked if he had felt the sick man's pulse, the sailor doesn't understand the question, but Morgan orders him to keep the patient alive, "until he should come with the medicine."

"The poor fellow . . . ran to where the sick man lay" but in less than a minute returned and "told us his comrade, 'had struck.'"

Morgan hearing this exclaimed, "Mercy on my salvation, why did you not stop him until I came?"

"Stop him," said the other, "I hailed him several times, but he was too far on his way and the enemy had got possession of his close quarters, so that he did not mind me."

At seven o'clock Surgeon's Mate Morgan visited the sick. Ransom reports,

> I assisted . . . in making up his prescription, and when I gave him the medicines and followed into the sick berth, I was much less surprised that people should die on board than any sick persons should recover. Here, I saw about fifty miserable, distempered wretches suspended in rows so huddled one on another that not more than fourteen inches was allotted for each with his bed and bedding, and deprived of the light of day as well as fresh air, breathing nothing but a noisome atmosphere of the morbid steam exhaling from their own excrements and diseased bodies, devoured with vermin hatched in the filth that surrounded them. . . .

Later, when the captain is given the sick list, he cries out, "Blood and oons, sixty-one people sick on board my ship, by God! Harken you, sir, I'll have no sick on board my ship, by God."

Morgan replies that he, too, would be glad to find no sick people on board but it is in fact otherwise. He has done no more than his duty in presenting the list of patients.

"You and your list be damned," says the captain, throwing it at him. "I say there shall be no sick on this ship while I command."

Morgan is later imprisoned as a spy.

Ransom's ship sails to the West Indies, where it is engaged in a battle against French shore batteries.

> When the cannonading began, the surgeon supported with several glasses of rum went to work, and arms and legs were hewn down without mercy. The parson assisting him, had the fumes of the liquor mounting in his brain [chaplains were also assigned to the cockpit] and became quite delirious; he stripped himself to his skin and besmirching his body with blood could scarce be withheld from running on the deck in that condition. But it was not in the power of rum to elevate the purser [also quartered in the cockpit] who sat on the floor wringing his hands and cursing the hour in which he left his peaceable profession . . . to engage in such a life of terror and disquiet.

Smollett is writing with the intimate knowledge of a surgeon's mate of experience, even if his personalities are caricatures and the events exaggerated.

Treating the Sick and Wounded

Ships of the line, carrying sixty to eighty guns, were provided with one surgeon, assisted by three to five surgical mates, all of whom were medical school graduates. A large fleet would also have a physician in charge who was assigned to the flagship and received reports of sickness and injury and issued orders to the ship's surgeons. A first-rate ship with a complement of eight hundred men also had several crewmembers assigned to treat ill or wounded seamen under the supervision of the surgeon and mates. Small vessels carried no medical personnel, and medical attention was provided by the captain and officers, who were eager to transfer their ailing crewmembers to ships with surgeons or to shore hospitals when the opportunity was at hand. When heavy seas and contrary winds prevented such a transfer, the captain had to make difficult decisions with no help other than a medical manual.

In 1703 nurses and laundresses were assigned to the British fleet and paid at the same rate as seamen. Recruited from seaport towns, these women often were the wives of sailors. However, women aboard the vessels caused discipline problems and were the source of much discontent and friction among the crew. Later they were replaced with male nurses, the reason for the policy change given by the navy being the predilection of the women for drink.

Medicine aboard Merchantmen

Most large merchant ships also carried surgeons who made the five-to-seven-month journeys to India or the relatively short journey of three to six weeks to the West Indies or North America.

When no surgeon was on board, the captain was unofficially designated as surgeon, and carried a manual of directions for treating medical and surgical emergencies. Crewmembers with minor aches and pains or colds, and even those suffering from fever, cholera, smallpox, or dysentery, were treated by the captain almost as well as if a doctor were present. The manuals described symptoms and listed what medicines to use for each symptom. Passengers, too, might require medical care from the captain, who had to serve as physician, surgeon, apothecary, obstetrician, dentist, and nurse. In the captain's cabin there were a medical manual, surgical and dental instruments, and catheters, in addition to numbered medications. Instructions read, for example, "Take number six for dysentery."

In a popular book written in the nineteenth century for the use of captains of ships at sea or other nonmedical practitioners on shipboard, fifty drugs are listed that had to accompany each ship, and the use, dosage, and preparation of each is simply explained. The second part of the book identifies common diseases, giving the symptoms and findings. Typhus or "Slow Nervous Fever" is caused by "contagion or effluvia, and its symptoms are languor, depression and fever with a quick, small pulse, vomiting of bilious matter, debility, and delirium. Scurvy is cured with fresh vegetables and acid juices."

Under midwifery, the assistant was to let the birth proceed naturally. The cord was not to be cut until the child cried and the afterbirth could be manually removed. The child was anointed with lard and then washed with soap and water. The child was to be breast-fed directly and given two or three teaspoonsful of molasses every morning. The book, easily readable and clearly expressed, would be a great help.[14]

Merchantmen encountered epidemics of measles, smallpox, dysentery, cholera, and malaria that required treatment. They needed help for wound management, too. Hostile natives attacked shore details, causing injuries. On one island the crew of an American whaler were gathering sea cucumbers for the China trade when they were attacked by the natives and several killed. On board the captain surveyed the shore with his telescope and was horrified to see the natives devour the bodies of the slain crew members.[15]

In whaling, many injuries occurred. Stove boats capsized, spilling the occupants into shark-infested waters; when they were pulled aboard they had severe, gaping injuries. The lashing flukes of a wounded whale could kill those remaining in the water. Captain Albert Wood found himself in a sperm whale's jaws. "The next thing I knew he had his jaw between my legs and I was sitting astraddle of his jaw, held tightly by his clamped jaws." He was rescued by his crew and treated for wounds, with one laceration down to the thigh bone. His crew gave him first aid treatment until he was returned to Tahiti where he recovered under the care of a French doctor.

The parents of a baby born on board a whaler had the captain identify his place of birth as "Lat. 36° 45' south, and Long. 119° 30' west." One seaman, recording the event, wrote, "Success to him, may he live to be a good whaleman, although that would make him a rascal."

Passing ships hove to for conferences on ailing crew members or to supply medication. A ship with a medical officer on board was a godsend.[16] In surgical emergencies, the medical manuals offered limited help. Tourniquets could be applied per the manual's instructions; bandaging and splinting for fractures were explained, and those assisting the sick or wounded could even do amputations as described—but with much trepidation.

The captain of the packet *Dreadnought* wrote a swashbuckling account of his own injury, when he was thrown against a mast by waves washing over the deck during a severe storm. His scalp was bleeding, his wrist was injured, and he suffered an open fracture of the leg just below the knee, with arterial blood spurting from the wound. He ordered his crew to apply a tourniquet and consulted his medical manual for treatment of the fracture.

Three members of the crew vainly pulled on his leg to reduce the fracture. He stated,

We tried to force the bone into place while the leg was extended; but did not know that bending the knee would relax the muscles so that the strength of a child would have sufficed. . . . I became so exhausted from the pulling that they desisted. . . . It was necessary for me to perform the operation (amputation) as no one else would undertake it. . . . I gave instructions for the taking up the arteries in case I became too weak. . . . At this juncture the second officer in whom I had much confidence . . . begged me not to amputate.

The leg was splinted and dressed and the captain was immobilized by wedging him into one side of his bed. Meanwhile, the ship drifted aimlessly while the crew installed a jury-rigged rudder.

Five days passed, and the packet signaled a French ship alongside. Unfortunately, she had no doctor, but the French offered to take the packet's captain on board; he refused. The packet arrived in Fayal in the Azores fourteen days later. After the captain was taken ashore, the local doctors told him an amputation was necessary. This time he refused to have it amputated: "A lone legged sailor is doomed to shore service." The narrative continues, "The exposed bone was positioned and held by wire passed through drill holes in the bone and lashed."

The most incredible aspect of this account is the fact that gangrene or a violent life-threatening infection did not develop after such treatment over such a long time period. He records in his diary, twenty-three years later, that "the leg is as long as its fellow and just as strong."[17]

Most of the surgeons aboard merchantmen were just out of school, with no funds or prior opportunities for practice. Most served for one or two trips and then quit. The tenure of naval surgeons could also be brief, but this attrition was not due to the surgeons but the policy of navies to discharge most medical officers at the end of a war—and then frantically seek to re-enlist them with the outbreak of another conflict.[18]

Hospital Ships

Hospital ships may have played a role in the naval battles of the ancient Greeks and Romans. An Athenian ship of 401 B.C., named the *Terapeia,* was probably transporting wounded soldiers. Later, the Roman trireme *Aesculapius,* which was attached to the Miscenum fleet, also may have been used for medical purposes.[19]

The Spanish Armada in 1588 included two hospital ships, the larger of which was *Saint Peter the Great.* Displacing 550 tons, she carried a crew of thirty seamen and a hundred soldiers, as well as a staff of fifty physicians, well supplied with medical stores. Neither of these ships ever served its purpose, and the *Saint Peter* was wrecked on the coast of Britain in the storm that scattered the fleet.

The first British hospital ship of which we have a specific record was christened the *Goodwill* and dates back to 1608. In France, the hospital ship *La Fortune* accompanied the fleet as early as 1639.

In 1664 a British hospital ship accompanied an expedition to the West Indies to assault Santo Domingo in Hispaniola. This squadron was defeated, and the only function of the hospital ship was to serve as the site of punishment for the adjutant general of the expedition, Captain Jackson. Jackson was court-martialed for cowardice, but instead of a firing squad, he had his sword broken over his head and was transferred to the hospital ship in chains to serve as a swabber of decks, the most demeaning job in the fleet.[20]

During the Second Dutch War in 1664, the *Loyal Catherine* of 289 tons and the *Joseph* of 101 tons were assigned to the fleet. Both were hired merchantmen. After the battle of Loweshaft on 3 June 1665, the *Loyal Catherine* accepted four hundred casualties, who were treated by barber-surgeons as she set sail for Harwich. Headwinds delayed her for a week while the wounded agonized and supplies of food and medicine were exhausted.

At the time, naval shore installations normally received casualties, but when none were available the wounded were treated in private homes and the government was billed for the service. Mayors of all port towns were to make provisions for the sick and wounded and provide surgeons. But the year was 1665, the plague year in England, and the terrified populace of Harwich refused to accept the *Loyal Catherine*'s human cargo. They wanted no strangers in their homes, and medical attention was thus further delayed or never provided to the wounded.

It was suggested that a plague ship be designated to hold the casualties in quarantine until the plague on shore had subsided. However, the concept of a holding ship, to detain crewmembers while their health was determined, was an idea that would not materialize for over a hundred years. James Lind, in 1754, suggested that the navy hold new impressed recruits on such slop ships until it was proved that they were disease free and could be assigned to a warship, but the Admiralty never approved the idea.[21]

After the *Loyal Catherine* was retired from service, ketches, doggers (small, two-masted vessels), or fire vessels transported the sick and wounded to the shore. Hospitals were built at Greenwich, Haslar, Plymouth, and Spithead. Later, Plymouth and Greenwich served more as retirement homes for disabled seamen.[22]

Other hospital ships were usually converted gunships, with a crew of between thirty and ninety-five.[23] Lord Howe's channel fleet during the Napoleonic wars consisted of thirty-two ships and included two hospital ships, the *Charon* and the *Medusa,* which transferred the sick to the naval hospital at Spithead. On other occasions that demanded a hospital ship, a warship would be temporarily so designated, but we have no reason to believe that they played an important role in this century. In most cases they transported the sick and wounded who were transferred from other ships to rid them of nonfunctioning personnel. The ailing sailor might recover and be returned to his ship, or he might die or remain chronically ill, in which case he was sent to a shore installation at an early opportunity. Some surgeons disapproved of hospital ships, believing that an ill sailor received better treatment on his own vessel, where he was known and was supported by his mates.

* * *

After the death of Queen Elizabeth in 1603, James VI of Scotland succeeded to the throne of England as James I. The English navy at that time was dominant on the seas, but the new king's first orders were to make peace with all his enemies; thus ignored, the fleet deteriorated. His appointees to the naval board were dishonest, and the administration, a sea of embezzlement, bribery, and corruption.

English ships in the Mediterranean were being attacked by pirates and captured seamen held as slaves. In response, James assembled six naval vessels of his impoverished fleet and ten merchantmen at Plymouth in 1620 to engage the pirates. It was with this fleet that the *Goodwill* sailed as a hospital and store ship. Although some sick were transferred to her, she did little good as a hospital ship and returned with the remaining ships of the fleet, chastened, and with their mission unfulfilled.

No nation during the centuries of sailing vessels was wholeheartedly committed to the idea of a hospital ship, but intermittently such ships were commissioned. The surgeon on a warship was expected to provide all medical and surgical treatment. In smaller ships without surgeons, the sick and injured were transferred to those with surgeons. The hospital ship, in any event, did not provide any additional level of care but accepted those men who could not carry out their duties until they could be returned to duty or sent to a shore hospital.

In modern times, hospital ships staffed with highly skilled medical officers and special equipment carry out treatment at a higher level than is available on other ships.

Ships of the fleet in the eighteenth century were converted to hospital ships by cutting ventilation gratings in their sides and installing partitions to segregate those with contagious diseases. They carried a staff of one senior surgeon, four surgeon's mates, attendants, cooks, and nurses and were provided with beds and sheets instead of hammocks.

Nutrition

Patrick Campbell, who served on several hospital ships, criticized the skill of the surgeons, the lack of medications, and the food: "[T]he bread brought the skin off men's mouths and so spoiled the gumms and loosened their teeth that they could not chew their victuals." The beer was bad, the flour and biscuits moldy and full of weevils, and the pork was overcooked to conceal the putrefaction.[24]

Nathaniel Knott leveled a salvo at the providers of adulterated foods and beer in 1634. "Little did these monster bellied brewers think of the watching, labour and miseries of a poor sailor in double danger of the fight and the shipwreck by day and parched with the heat of the sun; by night nipt and whipt with blistering tempests; and when he is wet and cold and hungry should not the poor soul have a can of beer to refresh him, but he must say 'mors est in olla' when he drink it, or a cake of bread, but he must think he is set to a penance when he eats it."[25]

It was customary for one individual to have a monopoly to provide food for the navy and for its hospital ships, and this position was very lucrative indeed. In 1705, it was decreed that samples should be submitted from several sources and the cheapest offer was accepted.

"Assorted Miseries"

In a well-run hospital ship, in which isolation of disease was practiced and cleanliness scrupulously maintained and which was provisioned with good food under the direction of competent surgeons, the patient stood a better chance of survival. For the most part, these benefits were not forthcoming in the age of sail, and the hospital ship was simply a repository for disabled manpower. The abysmal death toll at large civilian hospitals, where 20 to 30 percent of all admissions died from cross-infections and contagion due to the crowding of all the sick into a ward, was paralleled in hospital ships, until isolation was practiced in the latter part of the eighteenth century.

Between 1608 and 1740, about thirty hospital ships were in service in the Royal Navy, most for a limited time. About one of every five admissions died on these ships. One in five is no better than the death rate in civilian hospitals, but it should have been better, considering that the hospitalized patients were in a younger age group.[26]

On merchant vessels the chronically ailing sailor did even less well. Some captains intentionally abandoned sick or poorly performing crewmembers on leaving an anchorage. Robert Robertson describes rescuing an elderly man left in an African coastal village by a malevolent captain. The sailor survived for several months on the meager sustenance provided by the natives. He was treated on board before he was landed in the West Indies.[27]

Thomas Trotter was appointed as chief physician to the Haslar Naval Hospital in 1797, where isolation was strictly enforced and bedding and clothing frequently washed. The walls and floors were scrubbed with warm vinegar and cross-infection was held to a minimum. Trotter made some interesting observations about his patients during his tenure at this hospital.

He wrote about the despondency of these young patients, some no more than fourteen years of age. Yes, they were ill, but the youthful spirit was gone, conversation lagged, and no social relations developed among the patients. He attributed this to the horror of the patients whose next bed neighbor might be a seaman hospitalized because of brutal lacerations and festering sores at the draining sites of whiplash wounds on his back and buttocks.

Such whipped patients were so psychologically disturbed that they frequently went into fits of hysteria, weeping, and delirium, while the other men in the wards silently looked on and wept in sympathy, and finally turned their heads away.

At other times his patients came close to mutiny, refusing treatment and deserting. Trotter urgently requested and received administrative personnel to restore order.[28]

But his sympathies clearly lay with the damaged and disillusioned young men in his charge. Typically, he observed, a sailor had been born and raised on an inland farm, never having seen the sea. As a young boy he had dreamed of adventure in far-off places, and at the age of fourteen or sixteen, when the daily drudgery of farm life became so boring, he sought his escape.

The youngster would pack his belongings and head for the nearest seaport. Clever but never educated, he sought out seamen, listened to their stories, and emulated their salt-encrusted speech, phrases, and swaggering gait. Once aboard ship, he learned his duties by following his mates, guided by their advice, and as the voyage lengthened was accepted by them.

He traveled to all quarters of the world and knew no home but his ship. His life was centered on his vessel, so that even on his return to his native country his shipmates were his family. He had no desire for wealth but simply enough for a fling on his next shore leave. On shore he was unmistakably a sailor, carousing with his shipmates, to whom he was totally bonded. He would give his whole purse to a mate on request and expected no collateral.

The conditions of his work were often inhumane and it is surprising that mutiny was not more common.

John Milne, while a surgeon on board a merchantman, described the harsh working conditions of seamen. Under way, foul weather kept them aloft in wet clothing day after day in tropical or frigid weather. In port they loaded and unloaded cargo from the first light of dawn till after dark with one half-hour respite for breakfast and supper. In tropical ports they suffered malaria and dysentery, having barely recovered from scurvy after a long voyage.

Milne describes an incident at the dock at Whampoa, in Southern China. The captain was displeased with the manner in which a longboat was hoisted and stowed after his crew had been at hard labor all day unloading cargo. He ordered the detail to lower the boat and repeat the performance with more alacrity. Milne added, " . . . [T]here is not a slave in the West Indies whose labour is equal to that of a seaman . . . nor was their treatment more harsh."[29] The farmboy's dream became, as Rudyard Kipling described it, " . . . that packet of assorted miseries which we call a ship." The seaman's life was filled with dangerous and laborious duty, stormy weather, tropical diseases, and an unbalanced diet, all of which lead to premature old age and early death.

Yet when danger loomed and the decks cleared for action, complaints were forgotten and an esprit de corps surged through the crew, not shown

at any other time.[30] In a well-regulated ship even impressed seamen's dis-
affections disappeared in time, and bonds were made with his new shipmates. When an enemy was sighted, the bonds welded even tighter.

* * *

Without knowledge of the cause of the many diseases he treated, even
without knowledge of the existence of a bacterium, and without any specific remedies (quinine for malaria is an exception, as was vaccination for
smallpox) the naval surgeon proved his worth by reducing the mortality
from disease from one in eight in 1780 to one in thirty in 1812. Cleanliness,
improved hygienic practices, separation of the sick from the healthy, and
improvement in diet were his weapons. His pleas had finally reached the
ears of the Admiralty, and his recommendations were accepted.

Chapter 3

Battling Disease at Sea

CONTAGIOUS diseases treated by ship surgeons were ship fever, also known as jail or hospital fever (typhus), the gripes and fluxes (dysentery, which could include typhoid), smallpox, measles, and pleurisy and catarrhal fever (colds, grippe, and sometimes pneumonia or tuberculosis). In addition to scurvy and beriberi, food poisoning and venereal diseases also took their toll. In southern latitudes, remittent or intermittent fever (malaria, yellow fever, and others, undiagnosed) were also encountered.

The precise causative agent of these diseases was unknown, and there was no specific medication to treat most of them. Countless numbers of people died of smallpox before it could be prevented by inoculation and, after 1800, by vaccination. Countless sailors perished of scurvy before, in the latter half of the eighteenth century, they were supplied with freshly grown vegetables and citrus fruits. Beriberi killed thousands before it came to be cured simply by varying the diet.

Although battle casualties demanded much of the surgeons' time, they were insignificant compared to the morbidity and mortality of disease. Blane recognized the real enemy and carefully tallied medical statistics in the Caribbean fleet for the Admiralty. Seven hundred and fifteen men died on board, only fifty-nine of whom died of battle wounds. Another 862 died from illness in shore hospitals and on various Caribbean islands. English Harbour in Antigua and Port Royal in Jamaica were called the graveyards of British sailors. It was too hot, there were too many loose women, and there was too much drinking. The temporary shore hospitals in the West Indies were dirty and poorly organized. One person died for every five admitted.

There were twelve thousand seamen in this fleet, of whom 1,577 died, one-seventh of the command being lost in a single year. In addition, one man in fifteen was on the sick list, leaving about 9,500 capable of duty. He reported that most sickness occurred on the larger ships with two or three decks; men in frigates and merchantmen, where there were fewer people crowded together, were healthier.[1]

Causal Connections

The cause of all disease in the sixteenth to nineteenth centuries was thought to be toxic air rising from the ground in a miasmic cloud, or an effluvia of the breath of sick individuals, which contaminated the air and enveloped healthy individuals and sickened them. If large numbers of people congregated, someone in the crowd was responsible for spreading disease to others. In the absence of any suspicion of a bacterium or virus, the toxic air theory provided a reasonable explanation for contagion; the stink of putrefaction and filth contaminated the air and sickened people.

Toxic air in a ship was thought to develop under several conditions. With unfavorable winds, the surface water of the sea could sour, or if the winds were of gale force, hatches and ports were closed and the crew, closely confined below, inhaled impure air. The green timbers of newly built ships emanated odors throughout the ship that were also thought to be carrying disease. The rancid stink of bilge water and dead rats could also foul the air. To overcome these odors, ships were fumigated. Burning a tarred piece of rope, tobacco, or gunpowder was used to overcome the evil odors, as well as hot vinegar, substituting one odor for another. In an effort to overcome the foul air, commanders constructed wind sails, opened up hatches and gun ports when possible, lighted braziers between decks, and whitewashed the interior.

This was a propitious moment for inventor Sam Dutton to try to sell the Admiralty his ventilation pipe to change the air between decks. Dutton's large stove pipe, open at both ends, was placed upright between the lower decks and the top deck. Hot cauldrons of cooking food were set around the lower pipe and used to heat the air in the pipe, which produced an updraft, as lower deck air was vented with sufficient force to extinguish a candle.[2] Another method to vent ships was to force air through a pipe by bellows. The Admiralty was not impressed by either method.

The Beginnings of Disease Control

A ship on a long cruise was a superb model with which to study the epidemiology of contagion. When at sea, it was an isolated unit, not subjected to diseases introduced by strangers. Its crewmembers freely intermingled in close quarters. Sickness in such a unit would spread rapidly, but when the diseases had run their courses, the survivors were often immune; as long as no new infectious agent was introduced, the ship remained healthy.

Surgeons on merchant and navy ships expected to be busy with many sick as the vessel left port. Colds, venereal disease, dysenteries, smallpox, typhus, and the effects of drunkenness—the rewards of a dissolute shore stay—quickly became apparent, but as the days and weeks unfolded at sea, the surgeon had little work. (On long voyages, of course, dietary deficiencies might develop.)

This balance was upset when the fleet commanding officer transferred personnel to a healthy ship from a sickly ship; the healthy crew sickened. After a battle the vanquished, rescued crew of the enemy evened the score as they spread disease to the victors. Details assigned to sail a captured prize became ill from contact with the diseases prevalent in the enemy ship. In one instance, a child brought on board by its mother and fussed over by the crew started an epidemic of smallpox.[3]

Surgeons vigorously protested to their captains, and the captains to the fleet commander, about transferred crews from other ships. The protests were often not heeded, to the regret of the commander, as sickness weakened the striking force of the fleet.

In 1794 Thomas Trotter, naval surgeon and an Edinburgh graduate, was made physician to the Channel Fleet, which was commanded by Admiral Lord Earl Howe. The fleet consisted of thirty-two ships of the line plus frigates, sloops, luggers, fire ships, and even two hospital ships, the *Charon* and the *Medusa*. The total personnel of such a force was upward of twenty thousand men.

Howe, cognizant of the power of disease to weaken his command, instructed Trotter to report his health suggestions directly to him. Trotter intervened on several occasions to prevent transfers from sickly ships. With such support from the commander, Trotter was able to boast three years later that there was no disease in fleet personnel. Only four hundred men had been sent to the naval hospital at Haslar. Trotter bragged, "What town or village can produce such fine health as this?"[4]

Trotter was also able to abolish the traditional and shortsighted practice of demanding extra payment from the men for treatment of venereal disease. Before Trotter's intervention, one had to pay fifteen shillings to be treated by the surgeon for this condition. Thus, most men kept it a secret while the disease worsened. Itinerant quacks set up shops in seaport towns to sell worthless patent medicines, guaranteed to cure. Shore details were requested by those remaining on board to purchase medicines for them. Sometimes poisonous concoctions were brought back, sold by unscrupulous "healers." Some older sailors acted as consultants on how to cure oneself. Often the condition was not venereal disease at all but some other ailment of minimal importance, and the apprehensive victim was sickened by the medication.[5]

Scurvy, the ever-present menace to seamen, was given much attention by naval surgeons and many foods were considered to prevent scurvy. Trotter, taking his cue from James Lind, believed that lemon juice was superior to all others. At this time, there was no specific directive regarding scurvy. In 1795, when informed by Trotter that supplies of lemon juice in Britain were low, Howe empowered Trotter to purchase fifty bushels of apples, cabbages, and onions which were often successfully used when citrus fruits could not be obtained.

Admiral Horatio Nelson

Horatio Lord Nelson brought the medical revolution in controlling disease to the attention of the Admiralty. Nelson had spent much of his life in sickness, dependent on doctors for his personal health, and at an early age learned to respect them. As a young midshipman of seventeen in 1775, he was partially paralyzed by sickness contracted in the East Indies and sent home, his condition described as a "physical wreck." He believed his naval career had ended almost as soon as it started. Later, in the West Indies, he contracted malaria, which recurred throughout his life.

In 1780 he was given his first command, the frigate *Hinchenbrooke*, at an age younger than permitted by regulations. He was ordered to head the naval portion of a combined army-navy expedition up the San Juan River in Nicaragua in the rainy season, in the low-lying, swampy coastline where yellow fever was endemic. As captain of a frigate, Nelson was not required to accompany the shore party of marines, but he did, against all advice. In a few days the invading force withdrew; within one day, eighty-seven of the two hundred men in the invading force were feverish and desperately ill, probably with yellow fever. Nelson was among the 380 survivors of the eighteen-hundred-man force that had sailed up the river. Nelson had to be carried ashore at Jamaica and was sent home again.

In England he convalesced at Bath under the careful ministration of Dr. Woodward, who attended him daily. Upon leaving Bath and receiving Woodward's bill, Nelson protested that the amount was too little; surely there was a mistake. Woodward answered, "Pray captain, allow me to follow what I consider my professional duty. Your illness, sir, was brought on by serving King and country." Another physician close to Nelson in this period was Adair in London, who treated his paralyzed arm.

He recovered and was given command of a frigate, the *Albemarle*, bound for Quebec. Contrary winds and tempestuous weather protracted this voyage, so that Nelson and his crew developed scurvy. They were saved by an American privateer, which had previously been captured by Nelson and released. The privateer reciprocated by transferring crates of fowls and fresh vegetables to Nelson's ship.

In 1786 he suffered a mental depression and was again under medical care. Again he rebounded, and six years later he was serving in Corsica, where he sustained a laceration of his back and lost the sight in his left eye in battles near this island. In 1797 he was again under medical care with an abdominal wound received at Cape St. Vincent.

During the battle at Tenerife in the Canary Islands, his right elbow was torn open with grapeshot, and with a handkerchief as a tourniquet, he was carried to the cockpit of the *Theseus* for an amputation just below the shoulder. Two surgeons operated, and Nelson complained bitterly about the cold in the cockpit awaiting the surgery and the coldness of the knife blade as it incised his skin. This led to a fleet order that every cockpit must have a stove and that all instruments be warmed before use. Surgeon Eshelby, one of the surgeons performing the amputation, wrote an operative note, "Diagnosis—compound fracture of the right elbow,—immediate amputation just below insertion of deltoid—silk sutures to tie vessels."

According to the custom of the day, the sutures were left several inches long. One suture, probably tied around the brachial artery, also caught the adjacent median nerve, causing him excruciating causalgic pain and a continued draining wound until the suture fell out of the wound four months later, at which time the wound healed. Nelson suffered from phantom pain for the rest of his life, his brain registering the irritation of injured nerves as pain localized to the missing arm.[6]

In 1805 Dr. Leonard Gillespie was fleet physician aboard Nelson's flagship *Victory,* which was with other ships blockading Toulon. Health of the crew was superb, with only one man sick in bed on the *Victory* and an equally good record on the other ships in this fleet, although they had been on station cruising for over twenty months, with few ever having set foot on shore. Gillespie described how officers and enlisted men's morale was maintained during this length of time.

At six A.M. his servant called Gillespie and informed him of the weather and the course. He joined Nelson and his officers for a breakfast of tea, rolls, toast, and cold tongue. Later he spent the morning seeing the sick and consulting with surgeons aboard other vessels. At two P.M. a band played for forty-five minutes, and then the drums beat "The Roast Beef of Old England" to announce the admiral's dinner—a leisurely and sumptuous meal with the best wines, coffee, and liqueur that lasted until five P.M. The company then walked the deck, with the band playing for an hour. Tea followed, and Nelson would become very communicative. At eight P.M. fruitcake and biscuit were served. The admiral then bade his officers goodnight and was in bed at nine.

To occupy the men and maintain morale, they were provided with music, dancing, and theatrical amusements. Drills and activities occupied the remainder of the day. Health regulations, ventilation, and cleanliness were personally checked by Nelson. Gillespie's report on leaving the *Victory* pointed out how well health can be maintained over such a long period when the commander in chief enforces them.[7]

Mr. Beatty was Nelson's surgeon aboard the *Victory* at Trafalgar and his close friend. Of the thousands of seamen and marines in this fleet, only 186 were sick on that fateful day of the battle. At the onset of the engagement, Beatty, noting that Nelson was wearing all of his medals and decorations, tried to approach him to remove them but was prevented by the confusion on the deck during the battle. A sharpshooter, stationed in the rigging of the French man-of-war, *Redoutable,* spotted Nelson and shot him at a distance of fifteen yards. The ball entered near the epaulette of the left shoulder, traveling downward and to the right. Captain Hardy was standing near Nelson and heard him exclaim, "My back is shot through."

Carried to the cockpit belowdecks, where forty injured sailors were waiting for treatment, he saw his surgeon friend. "Oh, Beatty, you can do nothing for me—I have but a short time to live." He was insensate in his lower extremities and felt a gush of blood in his chest with each pulse. "I felt it break my back." He died three hours and fifteen minutes later, just as victory was won.

Beatty probed the wound but did nothing else. An autopsy later revealed that the ball had entered the left shoulder, shattering the acromion process, and had continued on into the thorax, fracturing the second and third ribs, then penetrating the left lobe of the lung and severing a branch of the pulmonary artery; then it entered the left side of the sixth and seventh thoracic vertebrae, severing the spinal cord and fracturing the right transverse process of the seventh vertebra before lodging about two inches below the inferior angle of the right scapula. Pieces of uniform were wrapped around the ball.

* * *

Nelson had a full understanding of the plight of a doctor on board. He wrote his friend, Dr. Mosely, on 11 March 1804: "The greatest thing in all military service is health; and you will agree with me that it is easier for an officer to keep men healthy than for a physician to cure them."[8] The means for disease prevention was at hand, but cure of disease was not yet a reality.

Because of Nelson's many encounters with doctors and his understanding of their problems, medical reforms in the navy finally became a reality in 1805. He gave his surgeons orders to provide up-to-date medical care to all crew members. In a letter to the inspector general during his last command, he wrote, "The health of this fleet cannot be exceeded. . . . I look to you not only to propose reform, but to enforce it." Finally, the voice of the naval surgeons was authoritatively carried to the highest command.

The era when commanding officers looked down upon surgeons as supercargo—a necessary evil—was over. Much of this new attitude was the result of success in preventing disease and emphasis on diet.

The number of seamen sent to hospitals was gradually reduced as disease prevention became widespread. Figures for seamen sent to hospitals between 1778 and 1806 are instructive, the percentage falling from as high as 38 percent to 6.4 percent.[9]

Proportion of Men Sent Sick to Hospital from Ships, 1778–1806

Year	Total number voted by Parliament in Royal Navy and Marines	Number sent sick	Number sent sick as a percentage of total number voted
1778	60,000	15,978	26.6
1779	70,000	24,226	34.6
1780	85,000	32,121	37.8
1781	90,000	23,812	26.5
1782	100,000	22,909	22.9
1783	110,000	13,577	12.3
1793	45,000	17,280	38.4
1794	85,000	19,248	22.6
1795	100,000	20,579	20.6
1796	110,000	16,860	15.3
1797	120,000	20,544	17.1
1798	120,000	15,713	13.1
1799	120,000	14,608	12.2
1800	111,538	17,747	15.9
1801	131,538	15,082	11.5
1804	100,000	7,650	7.7
1805	120,000	8,083	6.7
1806	120,000	7,662	6.4

Source: R. S. Allison, *Sea Diseases* (London: John Bale Medical Publications Limited, 1943), 177.

Chapter 4

Scurvy

BEFORE THE fifteenth century, ships timorously clung to continental shorelines, dependent upon dead reckoning for their position. Given new instruments for navigation and a lust for gold, though, the vessels of Spain, Portugal, Holland, France, and Britain began to leave the receding shore for long days and months. Their captains were undaunted by contrary winds, storms, uncharted seas, and hostile populations; such perils were expected.

However, new problems arose on long voyages, with crews berthed in crowded quarters and living for months on spoiled and moldy food. Diseases, previously little known, became the greater danger at sea. Often a vessel could no longer be manned, and daring expeditions had to be aborted—blunting profits as well as the spirit of adventure. The most pervasive and elusive of the diseases was scurvy.

Scurvy was unknown on the short voyages of the Greeks, Arabians, and Phoenicians in the Mediterranean and in the seas around the Arabian peninsula and the horn of Africa, where they made frequent landfalls. However, the Roman Pliny the Elder identified a similar condition, which he called *stomacace,* that he thought resulted from drinking bad water. Hieronymus Fabricius, in his "Antiquities" describing the history of his own country, Misnia (Messina, Sicily), reported in 1486 "this new and unheard of disease which spreads itself very much and not only prov'd extremely dangerous, but carry'd contagion with it. . . . The mariners of Saxony called it Scharbock, which in their language signified inflammation."[1]

In 1440 the vessels of Portugal started to explore the west coast of Africa, gradually sailing southward and rounding the Cape of Good Hope. In the South Atlantic they first encountered scurvy. Vasco da Gama, commander of a fleet of four ships departing from Lisbon in July 1457, finally limped into Calcutta in May 1458. The Portuguese historian Vieyra vividly described the horrors of the journey: "If the dead who had been thrown overboard between the coast of Guinea and the Cape of Good Hope could have headstones placed for them on the spot when he sank, the whole way would appear one continuous cemetery."[2]

With many of his crew suffering from scurvy, Vasco da Gama met some Arabian vessels on the east coast of Africa and traded some cargo for oranges, which quickly cured his crew, but the disease recurred before he reached India and caused additional deaths on his return trip. The connection between citrus fruit and a cure for scurvy would be a long time coming.

The Course of Scurvy

Scurvy is almost totally confined to the human race and the primates, although guinea pigs also can become scorbutic. The scorbutic syndrome is the result of the absence of a specific enzyme that converts gluconate, a form of sugar, to ascorbate. Somewhere in the development of our ancestors, a gene was lost or altered, dooming the human race to depend on eating the finished product (until the gene can be restored to our genome and we are able to synthesize it).

Normally, in human blood, twenty or more milligrams of ascorbic acid per one hundred millimeters of blood circulates throughout the body. In a human experiment in which the volunteers ate a diet completely deficient in vitamin C, the blood level fell to zero by the forty-first day. Surprisingly, the first evidence of clinical scurvy was not seen until four months after the start of the experiment.

Yet crewmen on sailing ships often showed evidence of scurvy by four weeks after leaving port, and sometimes sooner. Infection, injury, and poor physical condition are known to induce scurvy more rapidly; we may presume that adverse weather conditions and long hours of hard work also depleted stores of ascorbic acid in the body economy. Whether a diet of salted meats and stale water and alcoholism contributed to the early onset of the disease is an unproven possibility. Unfortunately, in addition to not being able to synthesize the vitamin, our bodies are unable to store it for long periods. Dysentery, so common aboard vessels, could rapidly deplete blood levels of vitamin C. Many of the sea surgeons writing about scurvy observed that it occurred earlier in the sickly.

The sailor ill with scurvy is miserable. "Nothing can be compared to a man sick at sea; the quarters, the lack of quiet, the evaporation and fermentation of the medicines, the air he breathes,—all combine to make him the most unhappy of the human race."[3]

The first symptoms are weakness, lassitude, and malaise, all of which were recognized by surgeons as early as Woodall (see below) in the seventeenth century. The first hemorrhages surrounded the hair follicles, particularly those on the thighs and arms, which were subjected to abrasive injury. Bleeding spongy gums and loosened teeth were noted next, then pinhead-sized skin hemorrhages known as petechiae developed; still later enormous purplish blue discolorations of the skin, ecchymoses, spread throughout the body and progressed to open sores or ulcers. Anemia was due to extravasation of blood but also to failure of red blood cells to form because of the absence of folic acid, which depends on ascorbate.

The material that fills all the tissue spaces and supports the cells and body structures is known as ground substance. This is the cement that holds the tissues together and was theorized about in a report by David McBride (see below).[4] Incorporated in this tissue cement are reinforcing structures similar to iron rods imbedded in concrete. These are collagen, a fibrillar structure twisted like a rope and embedded in the ground substance. Both the ground substance and the collagen are dependent on vitamin C, or ascorbic acid. Without this tissue support, blood vessels tear and bleed. Wounds fail to heal for lack of ground substance, and the collagen holding an early healing fracture dissolves, with recurrence of the fracture. Every organ in the body suffers. But small amounts of ascorbic acid promptly reverse the process, and as little as two ounces of orange juice a day suffices to supply it.

Travelers' Tales

The ages of sail and exploration were also ages of now-inconceivable misery aboard ship, especially for crew. Sailors lucky enough to return home alive left vivid accounts of their experiences.

Ferdinand Magellan left Spain on 20 September 1519 on his voyage around the world and suffered indescribable afflictions from scurvy. It took him three months and twenty days to reach the Marquesas in the Pacific, after rounding the strait at Cape Horn, and an additional month to reach Guam Island. Pigafetta, a crewmember, was the chronicler of this fleet. He recorded that food supply was short and the crewmembers ate rats and the ox hides covering the ship's yards, but that the worst of their experiences was that "the upper and lower gums of our people swelled so much they could not eat and they died." Only the wild celery that Magellan had collected in Patagonia allowed his crew to go as far as it did. In 1522 only one of his five ships returned to Spain.[5]

Jacques Cartier (1491–1557), exploring the St. Lawrence River for a westward passage across North America, had the unusual experience of having his crew sicken from scurvy while land based. Cartier's expedition wintered over on a barren island; unable to forage for food, they lived on the ship's provisions. A passing Indian party suggested that they drink an infusion of leaves and bark from a tree they called "Anneda," which quickly cured the sick. Later, the French naturalist Jean Jacques Rousseau imported such a tree (a white cedar, *Thuja Occidentalis*) into France from North America and called it *arbor vitae,* the tree of life.

Jan Huyghen Van Linschoten kept "A Diary of Occurrences" during his residence in Portuguese settlements between 1583 and 1588. One passage in his diary describes the arrival of the *San Lorenzo* on the Malabar coast and Goa. The captain had elected to sail from Portugal to India without having once put to land. Most of the crew were sick, and ninety had died. There is little doubt that scurvy had taken its toll.[6]

But captains were noticing that frequent landfalls reduced the number of sick. There was a connection—but what could it be? From the highest levels of admiralty to the most wretched seaman, seeking the cause and cure of scurvy had become, in a way, another age of exploration.

John Woodall

John Woodall served on several trips to the East Indies as a barber-surgeon.[7] He had encountered scurvy on his trips to the Far East, accurately recorded the symptoms in 1653, and even suggested the use of citrus fruit, among other medicines, for the treatment of the disease. Like so many other medical discoveries, his observations were lost, buried in the literature, before a new generation of physicians, a hundred years later, completed the circle, returning to his forgotten advice.

Woodall was an acute observer:

> The signs of the Scurvy are many; a general laziness, and an evil disposition of all the faculties and parts of the body . . . a discolouring of the skin with spots darker coloured than the rest, and sometimes also darkish blue spots. . . .
> Also itching and aking of the limbs. . . . Sometimes the legs falling away and

drying of the calves and swelling of the legs and thighs, discoloured into freck-els, stinking of the breathe, shortness and difficulty of breathing. . . . Their eyes a leady colour . . . swelling of the gums, rottenness of the same, with the issu-ing of much filthy blood and other stinking corruption, thence loosening of the teeth. Some have their muscles, yea their sinews of their thighs, arms and legs so wasted away that their seemeth to be left only the skin covering their bones . . . the cure thereof resteth only in the hands of the Almighty.

And yet to any man of judgement, it may seem a wonder how a poor miser-able man coming to land from a long voyage, even at the point of death . . . not able to lift a leg over a straw and scarce to breathe . . . , yet in a few daies shall receive the fullnesse of former health, yea with little or no medicines at all.[8]

Woodall described cures for the disease that included adding plants in the diet: spoon-wort (worm-wood), green ginger, currants, raisins. He also recommended "pure water, good wine and a fresh diet," as well as sev-eral lengthy prescriptions, most of which contain plant material. In addi-tion, "the blood of beasts," lemon juice, pepper, oil of vitriol, and various unguents were listed as curative.

Woodall also advised, "If your ship is passing a friendly coast, they should collect absenthie and juniper berries and boil them in goat's milk." Watercress, sorrel, scordium (a grass that smells like garlic), horseradish root, and bayberries are mentioned, but he returns to the bitter and sour (citrus) medicines and writes of the "juice of lemons, limes, citrons and oranges" as giving the best cure:

The use of the iuce of lemons is a precious medicine and wel tried, being sound and good let it have the chiefe place, for it well deserves it, the use whereof: it is to be taken each morning two or three spoonfuls and faste after it two houres. . . . In want whereof, use the iuce of limes, oringes or citrons or the pulp of tamarinds.[9]

Unfortunately, he diluted the credibility of this statement by asserting that any other astringent could be used. The ship's purser provided the lemon juice, and Woodall feared that if the purser discovered how good a flavoring it made he would use up the supply of lemon juice as a con-diment for the "great Cabins" (captain's mess). But no solely human inter-vention would succeed in overcoming this disease, he warned; "Without invoking the hand of God, no medicine will work. . . . These recited med-icines for Christian Charitie, I thought not amiss to publish, admonish-ing young men to be wise and careful to make right use of them . . . for the good of the sick and credit to themselves, and let them avoid slothfulnesse, avarice, envie, fear, pride, or what else may hinder these duties, that God give blessing to their labours and then the praise and comfort shall return to themselves, which God grant."

Meanwhile, in 1593, his contemporary, Richard Hawkins, told of the miseries suffered by his scurvy-ridden crew on a voyage from England to Chile. Hawkins, an experienced mariner, confessed that many of his long voyages caused death and desolation to his crews. He wrote, "And I wish that some learned man would write of it, for it is the plague of the sea and the spoyle of mariners, doubtlesse it would be a worke worthy of a worthy man and most beneficiall for our countries, for in twenty yeares since I have used the sea, I dare take upon me to give account of ten thousand men consumed with this disease."[10]

Another contemporary of Woodall's, Capt. James Lancaster, command- ed a British expedition to East India in 1601. This was his second attempt to round the Cape of Good Hope. Lancaster, in command of four ships, left England in April 1601. At 33 degrees south of the equator, many crew were sick with scurvy in all his ships. As the fleet sailed southward, more men became ill and many died, so that it was necessary for the merchants and officers on board to go aloft to maintain their course.

The ships anchored off the Cape after 105 men had died. The surviving crewmen were so weak that they could hardly throw the anchor overboard. In contrast, Lancaster and some of the crew in his ship were in excellent shape because "he brought to sea with him certaine bottles of the juice of lemons." This he shared with some of his ailing men, as long as it lasted— three spoonfuls every morning, and all food withheld till noon. This was a controlled experiment, the rest of the crew not receiving it. He thought the juice maintained health because it was an antidote to foods preserved with salt—specifically salted meat and fish, the staple of the seaman's diet.

Lancaster may have heard of this cure from Woodall, or from the Por- tuguese and Spanish, but it is not clear how he learned of the value of lemon juice in particular. Later, when he touched at Madagascar, he sought lemons and oranges.

Like most of the sea journals in this period, including Woodall's, Lan- caster's contained priceless information, the value of which was never rec- ognized in his lifetime. Thousands of lives were sacrificed in consequence, in the centuries to come. In his report to the governors of the Company of Merchants, Lancaster mentions scurvy but makes no reference to the lemon juice.[11]

An Age of Experimentation and Speculation

Experienced and observant captains and surgeons collected many anecdotal experiences, observing scurvy-ridden crewmen as they improved or worsened with certain medications, food, or living conditions. It was common knowledge in the seventeenth century that ordering a scorbutic sailor ashore for a few days quickly cured the disease, leading to the belief that the land itself had a curative effect. Each captain had his favorite recipe for a cure, variously recommending fresh food, an array of plants, wine, beer, exercise, dry and clean clothing, proper ventilation of holds, ship fumigation, avoidance of salted meats, and so on and on.

By then the Spanish and Portuguese were carrying casks of lemon juice on some of their longer voyages, but the juice was reserved for therapeutic treatment, not as a preventive, and was only sporadically used.[12]

John Clark

A hundred years after Woodall, the disease was still taking its toll, and another surgeon of an Indiaman, also employed by the East India Company, published his observations.[13] John Clark, M.D., surgeon of the *Sir Charles Hudson,* plying between Britain and Bengal, was ordered by the company to write of his experiences with scurvy. His 1763 voyage left England on 22 March and arrived in Bengal on 25 August. The ship carried 240 people, of whom 108 were crew, the rest passengers or military recruits to the British Indian army.

In June, three months out from England, twenty seamen were off duty because of scurvy. Clark treated them with wine, sugar, and various prescriptions that, he admitted, failed to improve the afflicted, and more cases came down with the disease. Later the problem was complicated by some men with fevers, a low pulse, and delirium. He isolated the febrile patients from the rest of the crew and the putrid fever, as he called it, spread no further. He was clearly able to make the differential diagnosis between this condition (probably typhus) and scurvy. While the ship was in port at Bengal, the scurvy disappeared, but Clark had to contend with dysentery and venereal disease, the penalty paid for shore leave and the cure of scurvy.

On the return trip, scurvy again appeared three months out, but it affected only the crew, not the officers, "because they had drier quarters." Thirty-three of his eighty-seven crewmembers were confined below. A landing was made at Madagascar, and after one month all the scurvy patients recovered. While on shore, they ate vegetable soups, pumpkins, greens, and oranges.

The ship also briefly reprovisioned at St. Helena in the South Pacific. Two months later, as she approached the English Channel, the second attack of scurvy on the return trip is recorded.

Clark's journal gives us a detailed clinical description of one of his patients, and his attempts to treat him.

> Joshua Christian, a young man of active disposition, on the 23 of June 1769 was confined below by scurvy. For some time before, he had been troubled with listlessness and weakness of the knees; and he became breathless and faint when he attempted to go aloft. His gums were swollen, spongy and bleeding on the least touch; his legs and arms were covered with small livid spots, not rising above the surface of the skin. . . . He was allowed extra rations, tea and sugar for breakfast and boiled rice and wine with dinner.
>
> With this diet, his symptoms did not improve, so a pint of fresh wort beer with sugar and powdered biscuit was given twice a day, again with no improvement.
>
> On July 3, his countenance began to look sallow, his teeth were loose and the scorbutic spots of a worse colour. . . . the wort was increased to three quarts daily.
>
> July 7: The weather was wet and cold, notwithstanding he continued the wort regularly, and his disease began to make rapid progress. His gums were livid, his breathe was very offensive and he was faint upon the least motion . . . , his hams were discoloured and he complained of flying pains in his arms and legs.
>
> Being now fully convinced of the ineffectiveness of the wort, two teaspoonfuls of lime juice were given three times daily; he was also allowed a pint of red port in his boiled rice.
>
> 20th July. Little or no alteration could be observed. As the lime juice was now finished, half a pint of mango shrub juice mixed with water and sweetened with sugar was ordered to be taken daily.
>
> On the 1st of August when he arrived in Madagascar, he was very weak and exhausted and it was the 23rd before he was capable of doing the least duty, although he was plentifully supplied with oranges and nourishing vegetable soup.

In spite of Dr. Clark's efforts, Joshua Christian's course was downhill, and almost certainly he would have died, a victim of scurvy, if the ship had not made a landing at Madagascar.

In the eighteenth century there was no prevalent idea about the cause of scurvy. To some it was poor living conditions, crowding below decks, wearing wet clothing days on end in stormy weather, made worse by continued work without adequate rest or sleep. To others it resulted from the month after month diet of salted meats, moldy biscuits, and stale water. Believers in this theory pointed out how rarely the captain and ship officers developed scurvy, because they had a greater variety of foods. Clark managed to obtain rice, wine, sugar, and tea for his ailing seaman, none of which were ordinarily included in the crew's diet, but it made no difference. Beer, especially wort beer and spruce beer, were thought to be helpful, but here again, no improvement was evident.

Why didn't the lime juice result in a dramatic reversal of the patient's condition? If it had, it would have made a lasting impression on Clark and served him in future cases, and the cure would have been included in his report to the East India Company. The probable answer is that ascorbic acid, the active ingredient in fruits and vegetables that prevents and cures scurvy, easily deteriorates with time, exposure to the air, or boiling. The lime juice or mango shrub that Clark administered could have remained stored for long periods on shipboard or may have been heated to the point where the ascorbic acid was altered. Although his treatment with lime juice was for a limited time, even a few days of treatment with a *potent* juice would have alerted an astute observer such as Clark to an improvement in symptoms. Such is the erratic course of the search for truth. Specific treatment was given, but by bad luck it didn't work, and the opportunity for discovery of a miraculous cure was denied.

Anson's Surgeons

Few recorded accounts of the ravages of scurvy can equal the horror suffered by the crew of Lord Anson's fleet. His eight vessels left England in 1740 on a course set for Brazil and then around Cape Horn. They were to follow the west coast of South America with the intent of plundering the Spanish settlements. The fleet was to continue across the Pacific to prey upon Spanish shipping in the Philippines and Asia.

The voyage was delayed in starting because of a shortage of personnel and equipment. To fill out the crew, he was given impressed seamen, elderly sailors taken out of sick beds in naval hospitals, and criminals discharged from prisons. Finally, after many delays, the fleet set sail on August 1740 but had to return to port because of foul weather. The account of the voyage was recorded by the chaplain, Reverend Richard Walter. In December they arrived in the Bay of St. Catharine in Brazil with one-fifth of the crew so weakened by scurvy that they had to be carried ashore.

This was only the beginning of a long series of misadventures set in motion by scurvy. The passage around Cape Horn was south of Tierra del Fuego, in the high latitudes; buffeted by severe storms, cold, treacherous seas, and adverse currents, they were carried back into the Atlantic when they had almost fully traveled through the passage. Then, scurvy again struck and half of the fleet's crew died. On the *Gloucester,* two-thirds died, leaving barely enough hands to sail her.

Upon emerging into the Pacific, a landfall was then made at Juan Fernandez Island (Robinson Crusoe's Island), off the coast of Chile, and 167 sick men were landed. Twelve died on the trip to shore from exposure. Even here, crew *in extremis* continued to die off for the first two weeks, while the remainder regained their health. Their diet on the island included watercress, lettuce, other vegetables, and fresh goat meat. Taking stock of their situation on leaving Juan Fernandez, the log shows that only 335 were alive of the 961 men who had left England.

Anson's surgeons described the case of a healed fracture in a sailor's clavicle that came apart when scurvy developed, the callus at the fracture having dissolved. The sailor had, in December, sustained a fractured clavicle, which was reduced and united. The dressings were removed in January, and he had recovered full use of his arm. In April, as he was suspending his body weight by one arm holding onto the rigging, the clavicle "disunited." At the time he was showing symptoms of scurvy. He was carried ashore at Juan Fernandez, the callus having remained in *the flexible state.* By three months of living ashore, he recovered from the "distemper," the callus firmed, and the bone united. (It is most probable that the bone was initially not united but was stabilized only by scar tissue.)

With his remaining crew, Anson captured the Spanish city of Paita and looted £30,000 of treasure at the cost of one killed in action and two wounded. Farther up the coast he captured the Spanish galleon *Nostra Signora Cabaderonga,* loaded with gold and silver, at a cost of two killed and seventeen wounded. Scurvy proved a mightier adversary than the sword.

Setting sail across the Pacific they repeated their error. On sighting Tinian Island with only seventy-one men not disabled with scurvy, they were becalmed for several days and, fearing the islands were in the hands of the Spanish, they hoisted the Spanish flag. When the wind freshened and they landed, 128 crew members were scorbutic and twenty-one died in the first two days on shore. Scurvy, not the enemy, wielded the scythe of death.

The two surgeons in the fleet were nonbelievers in the need for proper foods to counter scurvy. They thought that the disease was the result of sea air and that only by living on land could it be prevented. Three years and nine months after departing, they were aboard the one vessel of the original eight that finally returned to England.

On their return to England, Anson's surgeons discussed the scurvy problem with a Dr. Robert Mead, and all erroneously agreed "that the air is more than any other agent concerned in bringing on the mischief," although they admitted that diet played a part.[14] Mead had written that a bad diet would corrupt the blood but insisted that the air was the chief reason for scurvy.

In general, though, surgeons were in agreement that sailors recovering from an illness or in a weakened state from any cause were the first to come down with scurvy. A young, healthy sailor at sea on a regular seaman's diet in the mid-eighteenth century would not show signs of scurvy until after six weeks.

More Conflict in the Eighteenth Century

Sir Charles Wager, commanding a British fleet stationed at Leghorn, Italy, around 1750, was a convert to citrus fruits and ordered a chest of oranges to be delivered to each of his ships daily. The men ate the oranges, mixed the juice in their beer, and for diversion pelted each other with the rinds, so the deck was strewn with the rinds from which a delightful orange fragrance arose which "tempered the foul air arising from the holds."

But in a darker story from the 1750s, a fishing vessel from Greenland, at sea several weeks without fresh food, had a sailor so sick with scurvy he was on the verge of death. The crew put him ashore in a last-ditch effort to save his life, hoping the land—earth alone being considered a curative—would restore his health. He was unable to use his arms or legs and could not stand upright but crawled over the ground, which was covered with a plant that he ate to survive, " . . . grazing like a beast in the field plucking up the plant with his teeth." Shortly, he recovered. The herb was determined to be cochlearia, later called "scurvy grass."[15]

Captain Hugh Palliser, of the HMS *Sheerness* bound for the East Indies, was convinced of the importance of fresh food in preventing scurvy and, at the request of his crew, he provided extra fresh provisions instead of salt pork. On arrival at the Cape, not a man was ill with scurvy. The navy maintained that this good health was the result of a new ventilator system just installed on the *Sheerness*. To the chagrin of the Admiralty, it was disclosed that through an error of the ship's carpenter, the ventilator system had been kept closed. Moreover, on the return voyage, twenty-one were ill on arriving at the Cape, with the ventilators now open. Between the Cape and London, the original diet was given and none were ill. Palliser used this experience to advise his friend, Captain Cook, about scurvy.[16]

Despite such revealing experiences, the authorities, unable to fix upon the cause or the cure, floundered, and the conflict of ideas allowed scurvy's terrible ravages to continue. The House of Commons reported in 1762 that of 185,000 men in the sea services during the late war (against the French and Spanish), over 130,000 perished by disease and two-thirds of that number died of scurvy. James Lind stated that 133,708 men were lost by disease or desertion, and 1,512 were killed in action in this war.

The prevailing theories regarding the causation of scurvy by this time had become more specific but were not much closer to the mark. The causes included the sailor's continuous diet of salted foods, extremes of cold or heat, excess moisture and wet clothing, and unsanitary living conditions, including wet berths and dirty clothing. However, many attributed scurvy, at least in part, to the lack of fresh foods—that is, food freshly grown, not stored or salted food—but thought the missing ingredient was the "fixed air" in such foods. Some thought that fermentation of food was necessary to provide "fixed air," and most surgeons prescribed fermented malt or spruce beers: "In drinking a fermented drink, fixed air is thought to be released to counter the salted diet, moreover it is easily stored in a cask."[17] Because officers on board ships rarely developed scurvy, it was thought that wine, sugar, and other delicacies of their diet protected them. Thus, when a crewmember was afflicted, he was allowed wine or sugar as part of his diet. Woodall's prescription of "acid juice" a century before was lost in time.

Dr. McBride's Experiment

Research methodology to provide a single specific substance to a scorbutic sailor and deny it to another—the basis for our advances in biology—had not yet been discovered. Yet, David McBride in 1767 convinced the

Admiralty to permit him to give a trial of wort to scorbutic sailors in the naval hospitals at Portsmouth and Plymouth. The study was flawed for many reasons, and McBride couldn't get the surgeons or the patients to cooperate in limiting the diet. McBride persisted and had a second experiment made on shipboard, but no report was ever forthcoming. McBride's malt provided 0–1 milligrams of ascorbic acid per 100 grams, which was totally inadequate. (By comparison, citrus fruits provide 45 milligrams of ascorbic acid per 100 grams.)

However, McBride made some philosophical observations that related to the pathology of scurvy. He stated, "There is a principle in matter which hitherto has not been much attended to, and . . . this principle, forming the cement or bond of union among the insensible particles is to be held the immediate cause of firmness and perfect cohesion in those bodies whenever it enters the composition, and it is to be regarded as the thing that prevents their dissolution or decay." "Putrefaction" is the dissolution of this binding principle.[18]

This is an uncanny observation—uncanny because it boldly points a finger at the pathological basis for the development of scurvy. The collagen tissue throughout the body is a major supporting element present in skin, muscle, bone, cartilage, blood vessels, and the viscera, and this tissue is dependent on vitamin C, ascorbic acid. With "putrefaction" or loss of this tissue, the symptoms of scurvy develop.

Is it relevant to pursue the causes of disease by armchair theorizing? In McBride's case, his insight and theory were correct. However, until the cause of the disease was proven, they remained merely insight and theory, adding nothing to the *knowledge* of the disease. Moreover, McBride was well familiar with Woodall's references and quotes them frequently, but he failed to advocate citrus fruits for treatment. As William Osler, the well-known physician of the next century, said, the discoverer of a disease is to get less credit than the person who informs the world about the discovery.

Economic Impetus to Find a Cure

Increasingly toward the end of the eighteenth century, diet came to be considered a key factor in the causes of scurvy. However, understanding of the mechanism—the lack of a significant nutrient—was nowhere in sight. Until this scourge could be better understood and treated, seafaring was crippled. Commerce, naval operations, and voyages of exploration failed and thousands of sailors died. All maritime activities were curtailed;

improved ship construction and navigational advances were of limited value while this health problem persisted.

Observation and experiment continued. William Hunter, who had access to the records of the Board of Trade in London, which investigated the deaths of seamen, was able to conclusively state that crews in both cold and warm climates were subject to scurvy and that crews sailing with the trade winds, with little work to perform for weeks, or those on stormy courses who were overworked and lived in wet clothing for days on end, were equally subject to scurvy.[19] It was on record, then, that weather and climate could be ruled out as causes.

Meanwhile, however, the differentiation between scurvy, beriberi, and typhus fever confounded the surgeons and continued to make the diagnosis and treatment of scurvy difficult. Cleanliness and good hygiene, so necessary to combat typhus fever, continued to be regarded as a factor in scurvy.

Naval tragedies continued, too. The *Oriflamma,* a Spanish ship, en route from Manila to Acapulco, lost her entire crew to scurvy and other diseases. The ship, a graveyard for her crew, aimlessly floated the Pacific for weeks before she was boarded by a passing ship. Her misfortune was described by Captain Mendoza y Rios.[20] Yet in the same period Captain Cook, commanding the *Endeavour,* circumnavigated the world over a period of three years, making many new discoveries, with the loss of only one man to sickness. Cook made frequent and prolonged landings, and his ship was a model for cleanliness. In his log, Cook, acting on Capt. Hugh Palliser's advice, described his provisioning at stopovers where details were always sent out for fresh water, firewood, and greens.[21]

John Milne, Surgeon's Mate

John Milne, recently graduated from medical school, joined the ship *Carnatic* on her voyage to India in 1793 as surgeon's mate and wrote a series of letters to William Hunter regarding scurvy and other health problems.

The *Carnatic* planned to make a series of landings to replenish fresh food supplies at the Cape Verde Islands, St. Helena, the Cape of Good Hope, and Madagascar. In spite of these landfalls, scurvy still broke out among some crewmembers after three and a half months. As his published work records, Milne diligently tried varying the diet with spruce beer, wine, and food from the captain's table with a minimum of success. It can be seen that Milne's emphasis was now on diet.

Echoing the conventional wisdom of the period, he wrote that those in poor health, drunkards, and those with venereal disease and convalescents were the first afflicted with scurvy. In addition, though, he attributed a psychological factor to its development and course and often mentioned cheerfulness and motivation as an antidote. He noted that when a strange, unidentified ship approached and the decks were cleared for action, many of the disabled rose to the occasion with an esprit de corps not shown before that point in the voyage.

On his second voyage, no scurvy occurred. He attributed this outcome to taking on fresh fruit at each of the landings. The crew continued a salt diet, and he showed that this had no bearing in the development of scurvy.[22]

Differential Diagnoses

Toward the end of the eighteenth century, with weather and climate no longer regarded as a primary cause of scurvy, it was becoming possible to distinguish among the major illnesses aboard vessels. Typhus fever, with its febrile response, skin rash, coma, and delirium, was known as ship, jail, or prison fever and flourished wherever many individuals were confined in a small, filthy environment. Yellow fever, ever-present in warm climates, was diagnosed by the jaundiced skin and eyes. Catarrh and pleurisy occurred in stormy weather, when overworked crews continually wore wet clothes, and continued to be confused with pulmonary tuberculosis. Venereal disease peaked after shore leave and was diagnosed principally in the early stages, which were easily recognized. Beriberi continued to be confused with scurvy, although William Hunter did regard them as two separate diseases.

At this time, although surgeons had finally acknowledged that scurvy was diet related, just how it related remained unclear. Some thought it was an excess of salted meats, dry moldy biscuits, and an unvaried diet. Joseph Priestly had just discovered oxygen and shown it was necessary for plant and animal life; now some enlarged on the "fixed air" theory, claiming that stored food on shipboard lacked oxygen, which was found only in freshly harvested foods. Storage of food, it was claimed, caused it to lose oxygen. Others continued to believe that fermentation of food was necessary for a healthy diet, and beer and wine were still often used as a cure.

Amazingly, the *terra firma* theory persisted. In one experiment in 1775, some improvement was noted in scorbutic sailors who were buried in soil, except for their heads, and interred thus for several hours. This was a logical experiment if, as most people still believed, landing itself cured the disease.

But there had been more reasoned attempts to find causative agents. In another experiment in 1747 twelve scorbutics were transferred to the HMS *Salisbury,* housed together with a common diet of gruel, fresh mutton, and pudding, and divided into several groups. Group one had elixir of vitriol (an acid metal sulfate), five drops, three times daily. Group two had a quart of cider added to their ration, while group three had a spoonful of vinegar three times a day. One group drank a half pint of sea water daily; the last group had oranges and lemons daily. The experiment lasted six days, and the two sailors in the last group did best, one even going back to duty on the sixth day.[23]

In April 1794 the Royal Navy conducted another experiment on the HMS *Suffolk.* Each man received two-thirds of an ounce of lemon juice mixed with grog and two ounces of sugar. Seamen being suspicious of any dietary supplement, it was necessary to add the lemon juice to the grog where it was certain to be drunk. There was no control group. The ship was en route to Madras, India, and had no land communication for twenty-three weeks and one day; it arrived with no cases of scurvy.

James Lind

James Lind devoted his life to the Royal Navy and made many contributions to the health of seamen but received little recognition for his efforts.

At age fifteen he was apprenticed to a Dr. Langland, an Edinburgh surgeon, who was a fellow of the Royal College of Surgeons of Edinburgh. When war with Spain was declared in 1748, he joined the navy as a surgical mate and served for nine years. He then returned to Edinburgh, received his medical degree, and rejoined the navy. He was later promoted to physician in charge of the Haslar Naval Hospital at Gosport, Hampshire, which could accommodate 2,200 patients. During his first year at Haslar he had 5,743 admissions, of which 1,146 were for scurvy.

His first publication, *A Treatise of Scurvy,* in 1753, discussed citrus fruits and fresh greens among other remedies for the treatment of scurvy. This book went into three editions in English and two in French. In the following year he wrote a paper on the so-called Devonshire colic, which he correctly attributed to lead poisoning from orange juice stored in lead-lined earthenware (noting that the acid of the orange juice dissolved the lead).

In 1757 Lind wrote an all-encompassing book on the health of seamen, *An Essay on the Most Effectual Means of Preserving the Health of Seamen in the Royal Navy*. He described ship fever and related it to impressment of seamen with verminous clothing infecting healthy members of the crew. For this he recommended "a slop ship" to hold new recruits, where they were bathed and their clothes washed and smoked before they were permitted to join their assigned ships. This was never put into operation.[24] He also discussed filtering water in charcoal casks to improve its taste and lighting fires in ships to dry them out and to remove toxic air.

In 1774 his *Dissertations on Fevers and Infections* again discussed typhus, or ship fever, which he found could be controlled by quarantine of recruits and strict adherence to hygiene.[25] He also described the distillation of sea water to potable water, the credit and prize money for which, five thousand pounds, was given to a man named Irvine whose description was based on Lind's paper. Lind formulated an emergency ration of powdered meal and dehydrated soup that was also ignored by the navy. To improve morale, he suggested a uniform for seamen with a badge showing the name of their ship—a feature that was not adopted till 1857.

In the absence of specific orders from the Admiralty, it was up to commanding officers to put their ideas into action. Most commanders disregarded hygiene and diet as beneath their station. The greatest and most successful listened to Lind and other surgeons. These exceptions were the officers who established British naval supremacy, such as Rodney, Howe, St. Vincent, Nelson, and Collingwood. There could be no major naval victory without a healthy crew.

Lind's disadvantage may have been his quiet and reserved demeanor, his lack of pedantry, and his respect for rank and authority. His contributions to the treatment of scurvy did not specifically target citrus juices or green vegetables, but included proper air, good hygiene, cleanliness, and avoidance of salted foods as well. Discussing citrus fruits, he gives credit to the Dutch physician, Roussius, as the first to use such fruits in 1664. He makes no mention of Woodall, whose works he apparently did not read.[26]

In 1796, forty years after Lind first recommended citrus juice, during which time thousands of seamen died of scurvy, the Admiralty, prodded by another surgeon, Sir Gilbert Blane, ordered lime juice mixed with one and a half ounces of sugar for each man on extended duty after two weeks at sea.

What Took the Admiralty So Long?

The failure of the Admiralty to address the problem of scurvy, particularly after the publication of Lind's treatise, requires an explanation. Thousands of sailors in the navy were disabled or died each year. Even if the Lords of the Admiralty were insensitive to the humane problem, losing so many seamen each year created serious logistical problems of replacement. The situation demanded redress, and the Admiralty should have mandated citrus juices as part of the diet.

The Admiralty looked to the College of Physicians for guidance on such matters. However, members of the College were far removed from any experience with marine medicine. Traditionally, the early naval surgeons were chosen by the Company of Barber-Surgeons and controlled by the College of Physicians, who had no desire to minister health on board.

In their ignorance, the members of the College decided that any acid substance would suffice to prevent and treat scurvy, and, as oil of vitriol was cheaper than citrus juices, the Admiralty permitted vitriol or any other acid substance to be prescribed for scurvy.

There was one other reason. When Lind was promoted over many of his seniors to the position of physician to Haslar Hospital, he made enemies among some who had the ear of the Admiralty and who refused to subscribe to his treatment.

Lind had striven for and deserved success, but he never gained recognition during his lifetime. His counterpart in the army, Sir James Pringle, was renowned and made president of the Royal Academy; Lind wasn't even a member. Nevertheless, Lind had some allies in his struggle to convince the navy brass to provide citrus juices.

Thomas Trotter

Like Lind, Thomas Trotter devoted his life to the Royal Navy, but received little recognition in return. At the age of nineteen in 1779, he joined the navy as a surgeon's mate and rose in rank to become physician to the Channel Fleet under Lord Howe in 1794. In 1782, when there was a short respite from the colonial wars recurrently fought with France, Spain, and Holland, and the American rebellion had ended, Trotter was discharged and signed on as surgeon on the *Brooks,* a Guineaman, which spent eleven months on the Gold Coast of Africa, collecting slaves.

Trotter, who published articles on scurvy in 1786 and 1792, believed that scurvy was a deficiency of oxygen in food or water: Preserved food and water lost oxygen, became stale, and caused scurvy. He took issue with the then-prevailing idea that there were two kinds of scurvy, acid and alkaline, stating that there was but one scurvy and that it could develop in warm or cold climates. It resulted, he said, from a constant diet of salt-preserved animal food that lacked oxygen and could be cured by fresh vegetables and, in particular, with citric acid (which he believed was superior to lemon juice).

If his theory had stopped with this statement, we could believe that he had a fair understanding of the disease, but it did not. Like Lind and others, he thought the disease was caused by a variety of factors. He included toxic air from low, damp regions, swamps, marshes, and stagnant water. Scurvy, he opined—arguably mistaking an effect for a cause—occurred first in lazy, inactive seamen, and "skulkers" in the crew.[27]

However, it may have been in that connection that he related mental depression to the onset of scurvy. He noted his experience on board a Guineaman, in which those slaves who were mentally depressed on losing "their country, liberty and friends" were the first to come down with the disease.

The slave ship *Brooks* was picking up a few slaves at various points off the windward coast of Africa over an extended time period; they were being fed boiled rice, beans, and Indian corn. He noted scurvy among the slaves, but the crew had plenty of freshly grown food and were "immune." (Trotter was also wrong in thinking that scurvy could be contagious.)

To supply a diet of vegetables on long journeys, he recommended pickling cabbages, onions, and cucumbers to preserve them. Leeks and coleworts, cleaned, cut, and preserved with salt sprinkled over the top, were washed and dried and, after three months' storage, tasted as though "they were picked this morning in the garden."[28]

Trotter suggested that, while cruising in temperate climates, crews could grow watercress on a wet blanket spread over part of the deck. If wetted down daily and exposed to sunlight, decks could be covered with verdure. To prevent loss of oxygen in water casks, Trotter charred the inside of the barrel. Although he noted that the Netherlands Indies fleet in 1598 used lemon juice as a preventive of scurvy, he believed that all fresh foods were just as good. (He had no way of knowing that the Dutch practice of planting vegetable gardens and orchards at ports of call en route to the Indies—at St. Helena, the Cape Verde Islands, the Cape of Good Hope, and Mauritius—would enable them to colonize South Africa.)

Trotter suspected that Lind's method of evaporating and concentrating juices impaired its antiscorbutic efficiency. He stated, "Besides the water carried off by vapours from this preparation, we know not what other changes it may undergo by heat." (In fact, according to recent research, lemon juice prepared by Lind's method, by bringing it almost to a boil, loses 50 percent of its vitamin C and 87 percent of its effectiveness against scurvy after twenty-eight days of storage.)[29] Trotter introduced another way of preserving juice. He strained it through a linen cloth and put it into quart bottles covered with a layer of olive oil and sealed with paraffin to exclude air. The juice was then placed in a cool area in the ship. He reports that he used such a bottle of juice, which had been sealed for fourteen months, to treat some scorbutic slaves with the same success as with fresh juice.[30]

With pride, Trotter pointed to the health record of the Channel Fleet under his medical supervision. In 1797 forty ships of the line were cruising in or around the Channel, concerned about an invasion of Britain by Napoleon. The personnel of such a fleet would include as least thirty thousand men, yet only four hundred ill seamen had been shipped to Haslar Naval Hospital. The final success occurred in 1800 when the Channel Fleet returned to port after fifteen weeks at sea without a single case of scurvy.

Sir Gilbert Blane

Another ally of Lind's was Sir Gilbert Blane, who was physician to one of the greatest fleets in maritime history, assembled in the Caribbean under Admiral Rodney in 1780 in the war with France and Spain. He was Admiral Rodney's personal physician while the British naval forces were stationed in the West Indies, between March 1780 and April 1783. Blane reported a high incidence of scurvy in those ships cruising at sea but none from those in port, leading Blane to suggest that vessels be assigned to collect citrus fruits and distribute them to ships on patrol.[31] He was a strong proponent for Lind. Later he became a member of the Sick and Injured Board and, because of his superior position, he was able to convince the Admiralty of the importance of Lind's discovery and to provide citrus juice to all ships.

Captain Cook

Once introduced to salted meats, the sailor resisted any change or variation of his diet, so that the fresh meat and greens so necessary on a long voyage, when available, were often resisted. Captain Cook had to resort to flogging two members of his crew before he could force his men to eat fresh meats. Cook complained, "To introduce any new article of food among seamen, let it be so much for their own good, requires both the authority and example of a commander. I could name fifty instances to support this."[32]

James Cook, with a crew of 118 men, returned to England on the *Endeavour*, after a voyage of three years and eighteen days, with the loss of only one man to sickness, and this person died of tuberculosis contracted before the start of the voyage. Three other deaths were from drownings and a fall from the rigging. This achievement put to rest the theory that sea air was toxic and the cause of scurvy. Cook derived more satisfaction from his ability to maintain a healthy ship over such a time period than from his many discoveries.

The final entry in Cook's journal emphasized his interest in the health of his crew. "It is with great satisfaction and without claiming any merit but that of attention to my duty, that I can conclude this account with an observation which facts enable me to make, that of our having discovered the possibility of preserving health amongst a ship's company, for such a long time in such varieties of climate and amid such hardship and fatigue, will make this voyage remarkable in the opinion of every benevolent person, when the dispute about a southern continent shall have ceased to engage the attention, and to divide the judgement of philosophers."

Cook's opinions on health at sea were so emphatic that he was invited to present them to the Royal Society in London on 17 March 1776, under the title, "The Methods Taken for Preserving the Health of the Crew."[33]

According to Cook, there was no overt scurvy during the voyage, but Sparrman, a Swedish biologist who sailed with him, stated there were several outbreaks that were not reported to Cook.[34] James Pringle, the president of the Royal Society, wrote to Cook about the high cost of citrus fruits, and Cook replied that "although [citrus fruits] . . . assist other things, I have no great opinion of them alone."

Cook's failure to support the ideas of James Lind retarded the use of citrus juices, putting them in the background until Blane resurrected Lind's ideas. The methods described by Cook for avoiding scurvy and to maintain the general health of his crew include making malt into a sweet wort, which was given to those developing scurvy and those liable to scurvy; two to three pints a day per man. He believed this was the best antiscorbutic but admitted that it would not cure anyone in an advanced state of the disease.

He strongly recommended sauerkraut for scurvy and claimed that it kept its potency and could be stored for long periods. Analysis has since shown that sauerkraut provides 15 milligrams of ascorbic acid per 100 grams and would, if eaten in large quantities, be effective.[35]

Cook also insisted that his men have soup or broth with fried peas, which was issued to each man three times a week. Fresh peas provide about as much ascorbic acid as sauerkraut. (By contrast, a cup of orange juice contains 124 milligrams of ascorbic acid.) Wheat was substituted for oatmeal and served with sugar, which he also regarded as antiscorbutic. The prolonged and frequent stopovers with access to abundant fresh foods were indeed of value in avoiding scurvy on this journey.

Because fats and oils were thought to encourage scurvy, Cook ordered that all meat be heated to remove them; the resulting cooking grease was skimmed off and used to lubricate the blocks and riggings. Cook kept his ships scrupulously clean, scrubbing decks, airing holds, building fires between decks, and using smoked gunpowder to dry them out. Water was changed frequently, as he believed that fresh water and cleanliness are necessary to avoid disease, including scurvy, and to maintain good health. He even issued orders on the scrubbing of copper cooking pots.

He believed that the health of the crew was a commander's first responsibility, and he had the advantage of a first-class crew, all of whom were volunteers. He divided his crew into three watches rather than two, with no man on duty (when possible) more than four hours. His men were provided with extra changes of clothing, so that they wouldn't have to work long hours in wet gear, and he supplied them with special wool garments for the colder areas.

Whenever anchored, Cook had details searching out fresh greens and fruits. There was no schedule to meet, as he leisurely sailed from one coast to another, with long stopovers at healthy anchorages. Such a schedule in itself avoids the hazards of this disease.

It was evident that the diagnosis of scurvy was somewhat intertwined with typhus, dysentery, and other contagious diseases. Since scurvy was more prevalent in those debilitated with other diseases, Cook's strict sanitary measures reduced the incidence of scurvy along with the others.

Ship's Stores

The British victuallers in their choice of food staples were interested in selecting items that would resist spoilage on long voyages, were easy to transport, and would sustain life. The rations drawn for shipboard varied somewhat at different periods but, in the absence of refrigeration, salted meat was the cornerstone of the seaman's diet.

During the Napoleonic wars, the Royal Navy daily allowance of food was two pounds of salt beef and one pound of salt pork, twelve ounces of cheese, and eight ounces of butter for each sailor per week, plus ship's biscuits, dried peas, oatmeal, or flour. Four weeks after departure, the cheese and butter were rancid, the stores of flour and oatmeal were crawling with weevils, and the biscuits were so hard they had to be soaked in water before they could be eaten. Before soaking a biscuit, it was sharply struck with a hard object to drive out the weevils. Starvation aboard ship was not the result of food shortage but of spoilage. Water, which was stored in wooden casks usually in a warm storage area, became a reservoir for bacteria and fungi and was foul tasting.

In the early voyages of exploration, lemon juice is mentioned on the provisioning of Spanish vessels but not for prevention of scurvy. In the *Armada de Filipinas* in 1618, casks of lemon juice were stowed aboard. The Spaniards were also the first to distill sea water at sea, and this is mentioned as early as 1566.[36]

Bougainville, on his voyage of exploration in the South Pacific, provided his crew with a ration of 600 grams of biscuits, bacon, salt beef, cod, or cheese. The evening meal included dried vegetables in oil or vinegar; vegetables preserved in salt were reserved for the officers and the sick.[37] Bougainville's ship did have much spoilage of food, though. During one phase of their explorations, crewmembers caught rats in the hold and sold them for food to their comrades for five sous apiece. It was a fair trade; rats synthesize ascorbic acid, and thus they offered some protection to the sailors who ate them.

Dr. Samuel Johnson, the lexicographer, was quoted as saying, "A ship is worse than a gaol. There is in a gaol better air, better company, a better convenience of every kind; and a ship has the additional disadvantage of being in danger." To soften the hardship of the sailor and make the rigors of sea life bearable, a daily allowance of eight ounces of grog (rum), diluted with water, was issued twice daily in the British fleet. Admiral Vernon, commander of the West Indian fleet, introduced this custom to the Royal Navy in 1740 with a view to reducing the drunkenness of men coming off shore leave. However, this issue was so generous that many of the crew were drunk on the afternoon watch. An effort to substitute tea for grog was briefly tried in 1804 but was so unpopular that a general mutiny was threatened and the idea withdrawn.

At the close of the eighteenth century, knowledgeable captains and surgeons were convinced of the value of fresh fruits, greens, fish, and meat and, on long journeys, made strenuous efforts to procure these staples. Thus it was often necessary to sail hundreds of miles off course to a landfall where crops were grown and to store fresh food aboard until it rotted.

Various formulae were used to concentrate and store citrus juices, but it is likely that, in most instances, most of the ascorbic acid was lost by the heat applied to concentrate the juice into a syrup; the long storage of the extract, which is chemically unstable, further reduced its potency. Admiral Lord Nelson did not concentrate his lemon juice but stocked up with fifty thousand gallons of fresh lemon juice purchased in Sicily for one shilling per gallon before Trafalgar. It was said that Napoleon was defeated by lemon juice and the carronade gun.[38]

* * *

The era of scurvy first confronted seafarers in the fifteenth century and taxed the ingenuity of mankind to solve its ravages. Thousands of sailors died hideous deaths, voyage after voyage. The high hopes of explorers foundered. Naval task forces failed or succeeded, not on firepower or tactics, but on control of scurvy, and the map of the world was thus remade by those with the knowledge or the luck to deal with the disease.

The hopes of commerce and the dreams of empire builders came to be precariously balanced on how ascorbic acid could be obtained, preserved, and utilized.

Two hundred years after scurvy was described by Hawkins, "the work worthy of a worthy man" found ways to tame its malignant destruction, but the sea surgeons still had only a vague understanding of its cause.[39]

Chapter 5

Beriberi

I N   T H E   L A S T years of the eighteenth century, the dreaded menace of long sea voyages, scurvy, finally was controlled. Its cause was still not understood, but methods to prevent its ravages were effective and maintaining the health of a crew to endure long voyages now seemed a solved problem. The many febrile illnesses that remained were kept in check by isolating the sick from the rest of the crew. At this juncture a disease became manifest that had always been present but went unrecognized because its symptoms were masked by and included in the scorbutic syndrome. It was now necessary to reckon with beriberi.

The Symptoms of Beriberi

Beriberi takes about thirty days to produce symptoms; these are lassitude (often regarded as malingering by ship's officers), weakness of muscles, and accumulation of fluid in the tissues, beginning in the legs and working upward, flooding the abdominal and chest cavities and constricting the heart. It also causes numbness and paralysis due to its effect on the nerves, along with palpitations and irregularities of the heartbeat. Palpitations of the heart and tightness of the chest, with intense pericardial pain, allow the patient no rest. The brain may also be involved, and psychotic behavior may result.[1]

At the turn of the eighteenth century, the British Board of Trade was empowered to investigate overwhelming and recurrent illnesses or accidents of the crews of ships flying the British flag. Two ships in the England-to-India trade, the *Mornington* and the *Arram,* reported to William Hunter, the board's investigating officer, on illnesses and deaths on board during their long voyages to and from India around 1800. Affidavits were taken from officers and passengers.

Hunter recorded that the illness began with swelling of the feet that progressed upwards, often reaching the level of the abdomen and the chest; breathing became difficult. Some died within two days of the onset of symptoms; others lingered for weeks. Some developed paralysis of the limbs. One crew member was autopsied when the ship arrived in port. It was noted that his belly was filled with fluid, but all the organs appeared normal. In particular, Hunter noted that there was no bleeding from the gums and no livid skin blotches, the most recognizable and diagnostic symptoms of scurvy.[2]

Thomas Christie, Esq., Inspector General of Hospitals in Colombo, Ceylon, studied the reports of the Board of Trade and concluded, in September 1803, "I have no hesitation in pronouncing this disease to be the same disease which is well known in Ceylon under the name of Beriberi." He added that the disease affected both native and European troops. The symptoms of the disease were accurately recorded. There was swelling of the legs, then the whole body, with the abdomen being exceptionally swollen. Breathing became increasingly difficult, and a state of "Asthma Hydroscopica" developed. The limbs became stiff, and chronic fatigue and muscle spasm, along with a terrifying oppression and tightness of the chest, followed. Numbness and paralysis of the lower extremities accompanied an uneasiness of the lips and face, with tremors, vomiting, and cold extremities. There were protracted cases of fever and delirium ending in death, but death could come quickly, often in six hours from the start of symptoms. Christie had noted that the heartbeat was irregular and that fluid developed around the heart and lungs.

Mr. W. Knox, an astute passenger on the *Anna,* en route from Plymouth to India, left England in November 1799 and arrived in India on 11 April 1800, and later he described the disease.[3] After three months at sea, the illness appeared.

> The disease showed itself by swelling in the lower extremities, gradually mounting upwards; affecting the legs, thighs, abdomen. When it reached the thorax, it speedily terminated in death, the approach of which could always be foretold by what the patient described as a burning heat at his heart. As the disease was stated to be scurvy, I looked particularly for these symptoms and fully satisfied myself that they were not present. This disease seems to have been the same as that described by your correspondent in Ceylon under the name of beriberi.

The board investigated reports from two other ships, the *Porcher* and the *Scalely Castle,* which had incurred many deaths as a result of widespread illness. The symptoms described by the ship's surgeons and the officers included lassitude of the native crew, livid, swollen, and spongy gums, and a foul breath, as well as dropsical swelling of the feet and abdomen, difficulty in breathing, and often sudden unexpected death.

Differential Diagnosis

The confusion and misinformation attendant upon the identification of beriberi extends to its very name, which has been explained by convincing but highly disparate etymologies.

One recent work claims that the name comes from Sri Lanka and means "I can't, I can't," with reference to the patient's inability to rise at the approach of the doctor.[4] Christie maintained that in Senegalese *beri* means "sickness" and its repetition denotes severe sickness. (It possibly amounts to the same thing.) Others attribute the term to two Arabic words: *bhur* (shortness of breath) and *bhari* (marine). On the Pacific Ocean side of the world, the Dutch on Java called it "Nagasaki" while the Japanese called it "kakke."

But before anyone could call it anything, it had to be recognized as a disease unrelated to scurvy except in the common conditions in which they both occurred: long weeks at sea, a limited diet of insect-infested and spoiled food, foul air below decks, and the generally hostile hygienic and climatic conditions aboard sailing ships.

A single report submitted by the surgeon of the HMS *America,* a ship of war, in Manila described the symptoms of beriberi in a crewmember as far back as 1762, calling them an "unusual manifestation of scurvy," and this was cited by the board's consultants.[5]

Hunter submitted the *Mornington* and *Arram* reports to medical consultants who carefully studied all aspects of the problem, paying attention to the specific ships involved, the discipline on board these ships, the cleanliness, the weather conditions encountered, and the number and the condition of the involved lascars (East Indian crewmen). The report rendered to Hunter from these consultants erroneously agreed that it was scurvy, and—correctly—that it was not influenced by any factor other than diet. They disregarded the fact that none of the many reports on scurvy ever described dropsical swelling, paralysis, or sudden death.

Hunter disagreed with his consultants: he regarded the disease as a "suffocation from water" and maintained that it differed from scurvy. Hunter claimed that the two diseases did and could coexist, making the diagnosis in each disease difficult, "just as a body acted upon by two forces moves not in the direction of either, but describes the diagonal of a parallelogram."

On the *Porcher* and the *Scalely Castle,* whose Indian voyages were also investigated by the Board of Trade, lime juice was wanting. The surgeons aboard had recognized the admixture of scorbutic symptoms and had provided the crew with beer, sugar, and tea, widely recommended for the treatment of scurvy at that time. Still, the symptoms of swelling of the body and sudden death after illnesses of only a few days were not characteristic of scurvy.

The Board of Trade again pondered and reviewed the problem, unable to distinguish two superimposed diseases, and its report now went along with the consultants and concluded the cause of the condition to be scurvy. The symptoms of swelling, paralysis, breathing difficulties, and sudden death not associated with scurvy were thought to be, again, "unusual manifestations" of this condition.

Acting on that premise, the board recommended that every ship in the India Trade route stop for several days at the Cape in South Africa to provision with fresh fruit and greens and that salted meats be reduced; ports on the vessel were to be open for fresh air whenever possible, and ventilation to the holds be increased by wind sails. Decks were to be fumigated three times a week and hammocks to be aired daily. These were the standard recommendations to combat scurvy and infectious diseases.[6]

Identifying the Cause

The *Mornington* had sailed from the mouth of the Ganges on 23 February 1800, commanded by a captain and seven European officers. On board was a crew of ten native Portuguese and seventy-two lascars and Indian soldiers (sepoys). In July the ship was making way in 34 degrees north latitude in the Atlantic, just west of Morocco, homeward bound to England. Many of the native crew were ill, with swollen legs and bodies, and breathing with difficulty. One crew member stricken with these symptoms unexpectedly died, and a second lascar suddenly died in a similar manner as the ship entered the English Channel. After landing at Gravesend, the ailing quickly recovered without medical treatment.

On 15 December the *Mornington* was again outward bound to India.

Many of the native crew were again ill, but this time with fever and biliousness contracted from their land sojourn in a cold and alien country, from which they quickly recovered during the first weeks of the voyage. Not long after, the symptoms present on the inbound voyage returned. Bloated and swollen bodies and legs and difficulty in breathing recurred, and by the time they passed St. Paul's Island in the Indian Ocean, twenty men had died with these symptoms. When the ship berthed in India, fifty-six of the crew had died and the remainder of the Indian crew were so weakened they could not be mustered as the ship limped into port. Again, on landing, the crew quickly recovered, and it was particularly noted with interest that the malady was confined to the lascars and sepoys and that none of the European officers or the Portuguese crew suffered from this illness. Other ships reported the same chain of symptoms and the occasional death.

As other ships entering English ports after long voyages reported illnesses among the crew with symptoms similar to the *Mornington* and *Arram,* simple scurvy became an untenable diagnosis for this condition of swollen bodies and sudden death. Most diseases in the late eighteenth and early nineteenth centuries were thought to be the result of toxic air arising from filth and garbage and, on shipboard, from the stench arising from the holds of ships. The new disease was also regarded as caused by the exhalations of toxic air and from the putrid odor of the bilge water and decaying material on board, which spread among the crew; the treatment was to sanitize living quarters.

The holds of ships were cleansed, pursuant to this theory of causation, and when the *Mornington* was refitted, fourteen hampers of rats were removed from the ship. The stench from these animals was felt to be the cause of the impure air circulating throughout the crew's quarters.

The report to the board said that the lascars lived in an unsanitary way, wearing dirty clothes that they didn't change; this was regarded as a cause of the disease. The report noted that when the officers supplied them with clean clothes, they were quickly soiled. The official report of the investigation of the *Mornington* stated the disease was due to filth and unsanitary conditions and exposure of the crew to bad air in their quarters; deficient diet was also mentioned as a possible cause, and it was recommended that they have condiments with their rice.

Knox, the traveler on the *Anna* in 1800, commented that the cause of the disease he so accurately described was "a poor diet or exposure to wet, aided by despondency and mental aberration." On this trip some of the Malays plotted to kill all the Europeans; fortunately, their plot was discovered and they were confined. These conspirators, held captive, showed the worst symptoms. It was not foul air or uncleanness, Knox concluded, because they were confined in the waist of the ship on deck and the area was scrubbed daily.

Christie observed that native troops in the compound who subsisted entirely on rice came down with the disease, but Europeans, too, became ill in military operations with rice as a staple, if they had been in Ceylon more than eight months. He observed he had never seen a single officer with the disease, although they fell victim to other diseases just as the troops did. Nor did Christie ever see a woman or boy under twenty with the disease.[7] It was only after Asian crews were employed by vessels from Europe that the disease became evident; this occurred in the latter years of the eighteenth century. Asian crew members preferred rice to a European diet.

Some of Christie's information came from Dr. Ewart, a regimental surgeon, and was based on the sick register of the 80th Regiment of Trincomalee, Ceylon, for September 1798. This regiment arrived in Ceylon in March 1797 and showed no sign of the disease until November. Treatment—a nourishing diet, sea air, exercise, friction massage to the legs, liniments, blistering calomel, gin punch, cordial liquors, and tonics—was successful. Christie stated that a rice diet was a significant factor in triggering the disease.

Christie wrote, "I can suppose the difference to depend on some nice chemical combination which I have not sufficient confidence in my knowledge to explain. The want of nascent vegetables is the most common cause of scurvy while deficiency of animal food causes beriberi."

It is refreshing to note that the major cause, in his mind, was not impure air, but even his conclusions don't disregard toxic air as playing some role in causing the disease. "The system was debilitated by the particular diet made use of by the soldiers which is certainly deficient in nutriment . . . [A] sedentary life, and marshy vapors in the jungle contributed to it."

Dr. Halloway, an assistant surgeon in the local hospital in Ceylon, also discussed this condition with Christie. Halloway complained that the sepoys were sending home all of their wages to their families, not buying additional food in the markets, and subsisting entirely on rice. He requested of Christie to influence the government to distribute extra food gratis to improve the diet. In July 1803, before the extra rations were granted, there were twenty-four cases in the hospital and six deaths; after the extra food allowance, there were twelve cases in the hospital and no deaths.

Criticism of the diet of the Indian crews filtered back to London, and the East India Company broadened the rice diet with garlic, onions, ginger, capsicum (cayenne peppers), black pepper, turmeric, ghee (a kind of clarified butter), salted raw potato sliced with vinegar, and wheat boiled with sugar and wine.

Narrowing the Search

By the nineteenth century and well into it, beriberi was only beginning to be recognized as a disease separate from scurvy. It was still known to be endemic throughout Asia and on the east coast of Africa. Its frequency on long sailing voyages, however, was still commonly attributed to impure air and vapors arising from the timbers of the ships and collecting in the holds. It was argued it could not result from a poor diet. Why wouldn't a poor diet in Madeira cause the disease, if a poor diet in Asia could?

The reasoning processes followed in this period in pursuing the cause of beriberi took investigators down many blind alleys. At first the disease had to be sorted out from the many other maladies suffered by seamen, before it could be recognized in its own right. Moreover, diagnoses of the febrile diseases were at this time more easily made, and typhus, the dysenteries, and acute infections were becoming more diagnosable and could not be confused with this newly described disease.

The known facts regarding beriberi included its predominance in Southeast Asia and Japan, but it was also reported in Brazil, then under Portuguese control. If it were to be regarded as a tropical disease, why was it present in Japan? Why, also, was it more prevalent in boat crews and inhabitants living along the sea coast? The standard answer to this question was the cold and dampness of the coast and the hardships endured by a sailor. But this argument was also refuted; why then did it make its appearance, several months after the start of a journey, in warm or cold climates, in easy and stormy passages?

In Japan and other Asian countries it often occurred in the upper classes, who were presumably well fed, yet elsewhere it was considered the result of a starvation diet. One common factor agreed upon by all authorities was that rice was a staple of the diet when the disease occurred, and its exclusive use was associated with the disease. Another was that a crew-member, no matter how critically sick, would recover within a few days after going ashore.

Rationalization supported many medical theories around the turn of the eighteenth century and later. It was convenient to regard disease as the result of inhaling a substance in the air, except, of course, for a few epidemic conditions such as smallpox or measles. Even then, however, to ascribe beriberi to foul air required some mental distortions. Why must the crew be on board for many months before the toxic vapors from the hold affected them? Moreover, if filth, soiled clothing, and uncleanness were predisposing factors, why did the European crew resist the disease? Indeed, European officers, who lived in better quarters and in cleaner surroundings, were not subject to the disease at all. It was recurrently reported that rice in some way was implicated, yet no one had conducted any research on rice.

Much later, in 1880, the inspector general of customs in Shanghai wrote a detailed report on beriberi in which he accurately described the chain of symptoms and findings. Anesthesia and tingling sensations of the legs and feet were followed by swelling in these areas. The swelling ascended the lower extremities, and muscles of the legs became weak and paralyzed. As the chest became involved, the heart palpitated and murmurs were heard. Breathing became difficult and an intense, oppressive, searing pain developed over the heart. Sudden death was then imminent. The author of the report again concluded that it was the result of inhaling toxic substances and that its name—still subject to etymological variety—was given by a Malabar physician and meant a waddling, uncertain gait in sheep.

He also observed that it occurred in Japan, mostly in summer, and that the affluent, who ate better quality rice (milled) were most likely to develop the disease. Coarse foods, such as barley and beans eaten by the farmers, were thought to be helpful.[8]

In 1893, in a textbook of diseases of warm climates, there is a lengthy report on the symptoms and findings recorded after autopsies that showed fluid surrounding the heart and the lungs; major findings were noted in the peripheral nerves. Beriberi, of course—yet it concludes: "The action of some specific agent on the human body does not admit of any doubt. It cannot be the result of heat, cold . . . too much of one element of food and too little of another."

The author reasoned that if a poor diet in a non-Asian country does not allow the disease but one in Asia does, it is not caused by a poor diet. A ship that sails from a beriberi port with its crew in good health has its crew come down, months later, with beriberi. Thus, the timbers of the ship must have harbored the germ or virus or poison. He again absolves diet as a cause. "That a defective diet does not cause beriberi is certain; for if that were the case, the disease would be more general than it is, and would be the constant companion of famine and the chronic state of starvation in which so many Eastern people live."

Continuing, he asserts, "Another theory is . . . that rice eating . . . is at the bottom of the trouble, but rice is eaten all over the East. . . . People get better on landing because they are separated from the source of the disease and sailors at sea with the disease should be isolated from the rest of the crew." This was written almost a century after the disease was recognized![9]

However, by 1893 the search was finally getting closer to the target. People who had the disease gained weight, so it was not starvation, and it was recommended that adding wheat to the diet would cure those stricken. An enormous mass of literature on this subject had accrued since the original observations of Christie, but no one conducted a scientific study until the twentieth century, when it was recognized to be caused by a dietary deficiency.

Further research showed the deficiency to be thiamin, a part of the vitamin B complex. Milled rice lacks this vitamin, and an exclusive, unvaried, prolonged rice diet will cause the disease.

From the time beriberi was first defined as a disease separate from scurvy and the febrile diseases, the reasoning of the human mind followed a tortuous path lasting one hundred years before it settled on a cause and cure. It had to free itself of ancient and venerable concepts of disease, accepted by both physicians and the populace, that dated back to the Middle Ages and persisted into the age of steam.

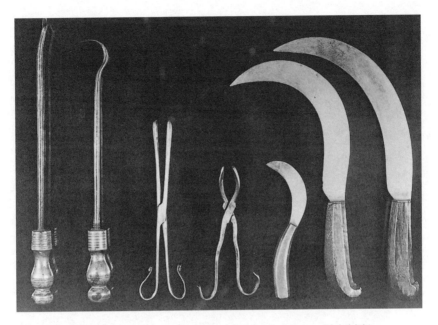

The barber's—and surgeon's mate's—necessities. Seaport Museum, Philadelphia

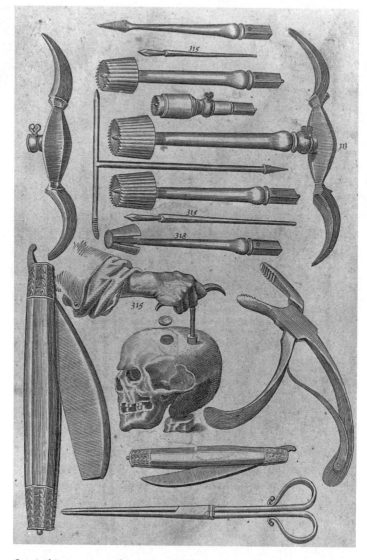

Surgical instruments, from John Woodall's *The Surgeon's Mate*. His concepts regarding amputation were far more conservative and reasonable than those of military surgeons later during the Civil War. "For it is no small presumption to dismember the image of God." Reprinted from Woodall, *The Surgeon's Mate*, 1655

The planets and the elements as medicine, from *The Surgeon's Mate.* All of these metals are poisonous. The privy council of the city of Westminster gave Woodall a medal for a pill that he prescribed that was said to have saved sixty people afflicted by the plague in 1638. Reprinted from Woodall, *The Surgeon's Mate*, 1655

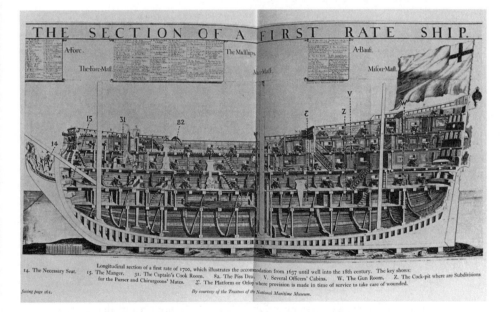

THE SECTION OF A FIRST RATE SHIP.

A-Fore. The Midships. A-Baft.
The Fore-Mast. Main-Mast. Mison-Mast.

14. The Necessary Seat.   Longitudinal section of a first rate of 1700, which illustrates the accommodation from 1637 until well into the 18th century. The key shows: 15. The Manger.   31. The Captain's Cook Room.   82. The Piss Dale.   V. Several Officers' Cabins.   W. The Gun Room.   Z. The Cock-pit where are Subdivisions for the Purser and Chirurgeons' Mates.   ꞩ. The Platform or Orlop where provision is made in time of service to take care of wounded.

facing page 161.   By courtesy of the Trustees of the National Maritime Museum.

Cross section of a typical British warship, 1700–1850. A first-rate ship, with a complement of eight hundred men, also had several crewmembers assigned to treat ill or wounded seamen under the supervision of the surgeon and mates. Small vessels carried no medical personnel. National Maritime Museum, Greenwich

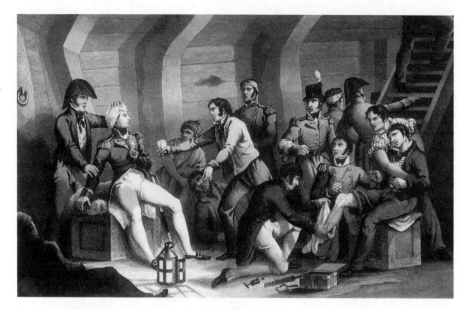

Wounded Nelson at the Battle of the Nile. Nelson spent much of his life in sickness, dependent on doctors for his personal health, and at an early age had learned to respect them. National Archives of Medicine, Washington, D.C.

The amputation of Nelson's arm aboard the *Theseus,* as documented by the surgeon's log. During the battle at Tenerife in the Canary Islands, Nelson's right elbow was torn open with grapeshot, and with a handkerchief as a tourniquet, he was carried to the cockpit of the *Theseus* for an amputation just below the shoulder. Public Record Office, London

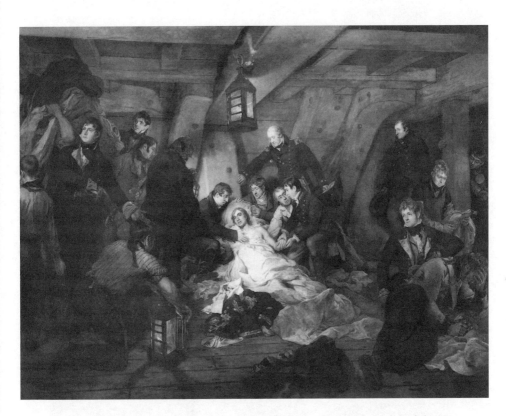

Dr. Beatty and the surgeon's mate, Mr. Smith, flank the dying Nelson aboard the *Victory*, while Lieutenant Bligh (later of *Bounty* fame) and others attend. Carried to the cockpit where forty injured sailors were waiting for treatment, Nelson saw his surgeon friend. "Oh, Beatty, you can do nothing for me—I have but a short time to live." He died two hours and forty-five minutes later, just as victory was won. National Maritime Museum, Greenwich

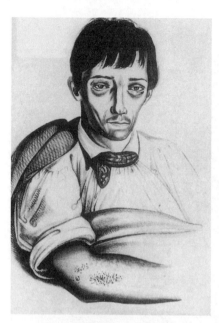

A scorbutic sailor. The first hemorrhages surrounded the hair follicles, particularly those on thighs and arms that were subjected to abrasive injury. Bleeding, spongy gums and loosened teeth were noticed next, then pinhead-sized skin hemorrhages known as petechiae developed. Still later enormous purplish blue discolorations of the skin, ecchymoses, spread throughout the body. National Archives of Medicine, Washington, D.C.

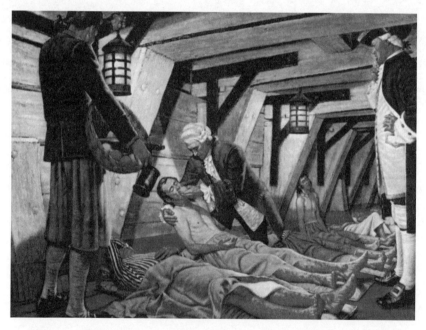

Lind attends a scorbutic sailor while skeptical attendants watch. Lind's disadvantage may have been his quiet and reserved demeanor, his lack of pedantry, and his respect for rank and authority. Forty years after Lind first recommended citrus juice, during which time thousands of seamen died of scurvy, the Admiralty ordered lime juice for each man on extended duty after two weeks at sea. Parke Davis, division of Warner Lambert Pharmaceuticals

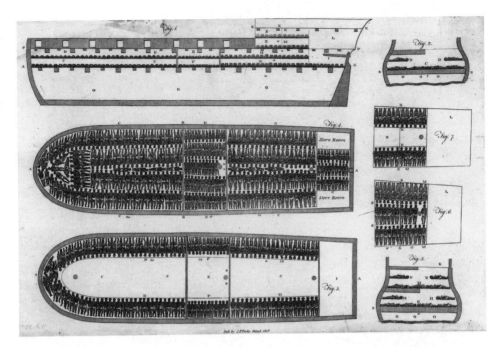

Occupancy plan for a slave ship, 1808. The figures for the number of slaves transported in these ships and the deaths during transport were supplied by the various surgeons and certified under oath to the customs officers at the debarkation points. The average number carried per ship was two hundred slaves. Library Co. of Philadelphia

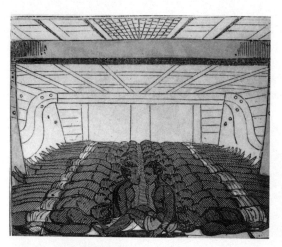

Looking into the hold of a slave ship. When the ship began the transatlantic crossing, the victims were removed from the deck and herded below into the hold, chained in pairs. National Maritime Museum, Greenwich

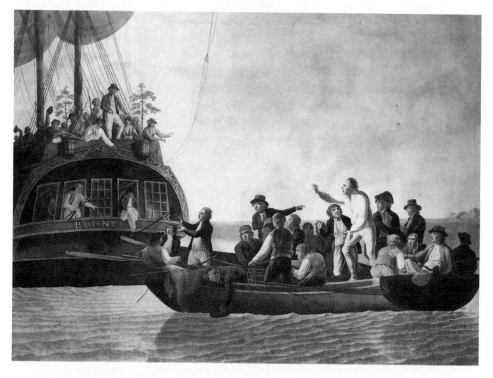

Mutineers force Bligh off the *Bounty* in a longboat. Survivorship is well recorded on one of the longest trips in an open boat, by Capt. William Bligh of the HMS *Bounty*, sailing in a launch twenty-three feet long with a beam of six feet, nine inches, which was crowded and low in the water with eighteen seamen, from Tafoa, near Tahiti, to the island of Timor in Indonesia, a distance of 3,618 miles over a period of forty-one days. National Maritime Museum, Greenwich

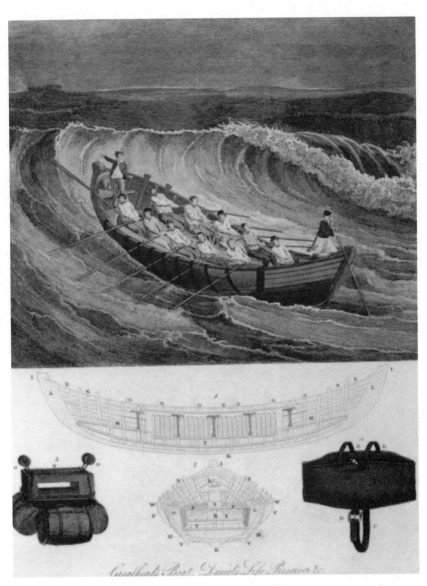

Mr. Greathead's lifeboat and life preserver. The first lifeboat to rescue a survivor was a boat planned and constructed by a landlubber named Greathead and launched in 1790. By 1803 Greathead had built thirty-one such rescue boats. Free Library of Philadelphia

CONTENTS OF A MEDICINE CHEST.

PROPORTIONS ACCORDING TO THE NUMBER OF PERSONS IN A SHIP, AND THE FAIR PRICE OF EACH MEDICINE.

NO.	NAMES.	From 16 to 40 men. lb. oz.	$ cts.	From 8 to 16 men. lb. oz.	$ cts.	Less than 8 men. lb. oz.	$ cts.	DOSES INTERNALLY GIVEN.
1	Alum.	4	6	2	4	1	3	4 grs. of powder, made into a pill.
	Ammonia. See Hartshorn.							
2	Antimony (or Tartar Emetic), in 4 grain powders, for emetics and solutions; also for cough and fever mixtures, &c. No. 50, 30, and 20, according to No. of men.		35		25		15	Dissolve each in 4 table-spoonfuls of warm water.
3	Balsam Copaiva.	8	60	8	60	4	40	20 drops on sugar or water.
4	Blister Plaster. (In roll.)	6	55	3	30	2	20	
5	Blue Pill. (In mass.)	4	35	2	20	1	12	One pill for syphilis; four as a cathartic.
6	Blue Vitriol.	½	4	½	4	½	4	As an emetic in case of swallowed poison, 15 grs. in a glass of water.
7	Calomel Pills,2 grs.each,No. 200, 100, 80. (Tin box.)	1	50		80		70	1 or 2, morning and evening, insyphilis.
8	Calomel.	1	20	½	15	½	12	20 to 30 grs. for a cathartic in malignant fevers, and cholera of India, and the West Indies, and Africa.
9	Calomel & Jalap Powders,10 grs. each, No. 40, 25, 10.		50		30		20	
10	Camomile Flowers. (Box.)	8	30	4	17	2	10	
11	Castor Oil.	1	30	8	20	6	15	One to three table-spoonfuls.
12	Camphor, Spts.	1	50	8	30	6	25	A tea-spoonful.
13	Caustic.	½	25	½	25	½	25	

NOTES AND DIRECTIONS CONCERNING EACH MEDICINE.

No. 1 Is chiefly useful externally to stop bleeding, and for fungous ulcers; for gargles for sore throat, by dissolving a tea-spoonful in a tumbler of water. Internally, in obstinate diarrhœa, in pills.

2 As an emetic take one table-spoonful every 15 minutes, until it vomits. In lung fever and pleurisy, and other high inflammations, two tea-spoonfuls. In coughs and fevers, one tea-spoonful. See " Pectoral " and " Cooling Mixture," in the Appendix.

3 Balsam Copaiva, given chiefly for gonorrhœa, and gleet; dose 20 drops, three times a day, dropped on the surface of a glass of water, or into sugar. It is good in piles.

4 Useful in local pains and inflammations, particularly about the lungs; may be spread on cloth or leather, very thin, and applied near the part affected, and allowed to remain twelve hours.

5 Useful in biliary obstructions, especially after having had bilious fevers in tropical climates. Also in syphilis, morning and evening, in doses of 3 or 4 grs. When taken as a cathartic, it should be followed soon after with other physic to assist its operation.

6 Useful to touch old ulcers with; a solution of it may be drawn into the nose when bleeding; sometimes given as an emetic.

7 May be taken night and morning, in cases of syphilis that absolutely require it. Most recent cases can be cured without mercury.

8 In the fevers and fluxes of India, Western Africa, and the West Indies, large doses of 10 to 20 grains are given at the onset of the disease, and salivation is hastened by frequent small doses.

9 Given when very strong cathartics are required, as in brain fever, and commencing jaundice.

10 Useful in a recovery from fever, and in other cases of debility. Made like other herb teas.

11 Several extra bottles of this should be taken on long voyages. A tin canister is safer at sea.

12 The gum loses fast by evaporation. It is best to mix it in less spirit than will dissolve it, and replenish the bottle with spirit. It is a useful medicine in typhus fever, and for colics. Also for liniments, for rheumatism, mixed with olive oil and ammonia, equal parts.

13 This is chiefly used to touch chancres with.

"Contents of a Medicine Chest," from a U.S. ship's medical manual, 1851. In the captain's cabin of U.S. merchant ships, a medical guide book was second in importance only to the table of navigation and charts.

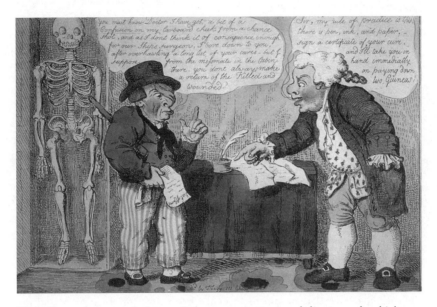

The sailor and the quack doctor. Sailors reporting venereal disease to the ship's surgeons were fined, so they sought treatment ashore. National Archives of Medicine, Washington, D.C.

THE ENTERPRISING DOCTOR

The Seaman said, "You must know, doctor, I have a bit of confusion on my larboard cheek from a chance shot, and as I don't think it is of consequence enough for our ship's surgeon, I bore down to you after overhauling a long list of your cures but I suppose from the messmates in the cabin that you don't always make a return of the killed and wounded?"

The Doctor said, "Sir, my rule of practice is this: There is a pen, ink, and paper; sign a certificate of your cure and I'll take you in hand immediately on paying down two guineas."

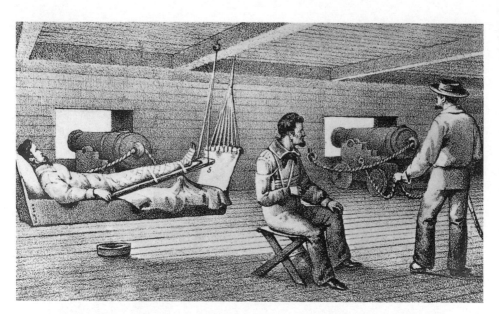

Injured sailor aboard a U.S. Navy ship. After treatment, patients were removed from the cockpit to the adjacent gun room or the berth deck for observation, and the slightly wounded were ordered back to duty. Seaport Museum of Philadelphia

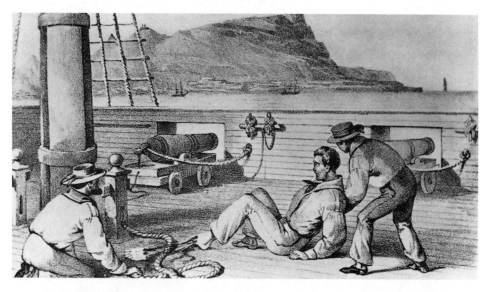

An accident aboard a U.S. ship. Of the 488 sick visits listed in the daybook by surgeon St. Medard, 6 percent were for injuries, including falls from rigging resulting in fractures and dislocations. Seaport Museum of Philadelphia

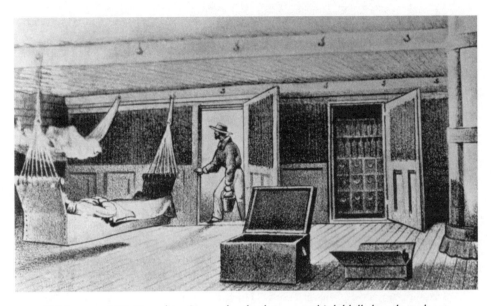

Sick bay on a U.S. Navy ship. Once a day the doctor sent his loblolly boy throughout the ship ringing a bell to advertise that he was having sick call. After this he attended those in the sick berth and made two lists of those who were excused from duty; one was given to the captain, the other was sent to the binnacle for the officer of the day.
Seaport Museum of Philadelphia

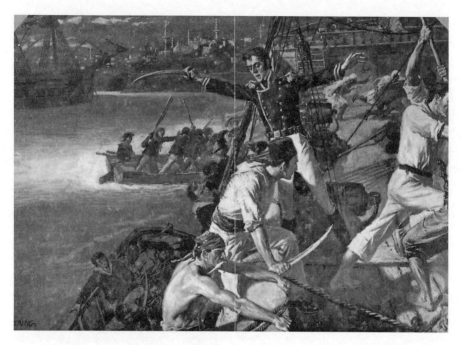

Decatur outwits the pirates at Tripoli. During the night, Lt. Stephen Decatur, with a commando crew, had boarded the *Philadelphia* and succeeded in setting her afire. Nelson called Decatur's action "the most bold and daring of the age." Library of Congress

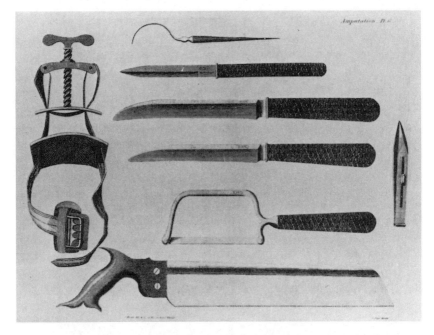

Amputation knives in use in the colonies. In the United States in 1709, a law mandated that every vessel carry a medicine chest provided by a competent apothecary and accompanied by a medical manual. For surgery, bandages and splints were to be stocked, as well as catheters, syringes, and a small knife for bleeding; larger knives for making incisions and amputation knives and saws, in addition to needles and thread for closing wounds, were listed. Reprinted from Turnbull, *The Naval Surgeon,* 1806

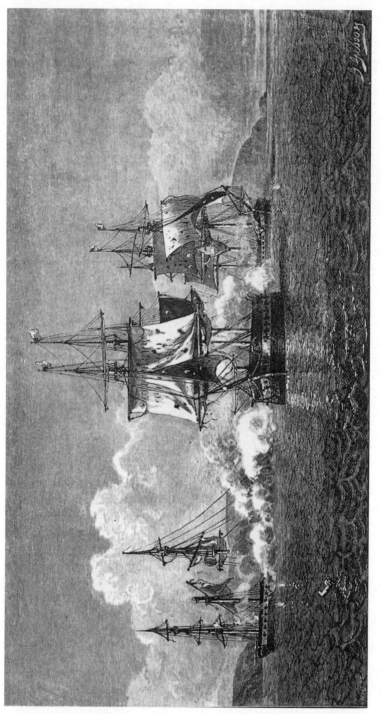

The *Essex* joins the *Phoebe* and the *Cherub* in battle. David Glasgow Farragut was the captain's aide as the *Essex* dueled with British frigates *Phoebe* and *Cherub*. Library Co. of Philadelphia

Chapter 6

Typhus and Tropical Fevers

S O ENTRENCHED in conventional wisdom was the threat of bad air, and so accustomed the population to vermin of all kinds, at sea and on land, that the evidence against the latter as vectors of disease was ignored for centuries. Since malodorous air and insects commonly occurred together, the best minds of the times could draw no firm conclusions.

Typhus

Typhus has accompanied the armies and navies of the world from the most ancient times. In the eighteenth and in the nineteenth centuries typhus was variously known as jail, hospital, army, or ship fever, and each was thought to arise from the stench of soiled clothing. In fact, the causative rickettsiae are carried by infected body lice or fleas. Lice and fleas are both wingless, parasitic, blood-sucking insects (the latter distinguished by its jumping behavior) that thrive in filthy clothing and bedding. The fleas carried by ever-present rats aboard ship were vectors for bubonic plague as well as typhus.

All ships were infested with rats that fed on and spoiled stored food supplies. For that reason alone and long before rats were associated with typhus, navies sought the services of rat-catchers. Rat-catchers were employed on ships in the victualing stations and shipyards. Thomas Swayne enjoyed a reputation as a rat-catcher and, in 1773, claimed a world record for rats caught in a single ship, HMS *Duke,* having caught 2,475 rats on board. His method of killing the rats was to roll up arsenic in a flour ball.

Symptoms of Typhus

As early as 1697, William Cockborn described a typhus-infected ship. As surgeon on board HMS *Duchess,* he described widespread sickness of the crew.

> This ship was the most sickly in the fleet, and had in the time of my abode above one hundred of these Sick Persons whom I visited once every day. The first Period of the fever was in the space of twelve hours; commonly, they were furiously delirious—they had a great pulse and Died in three days, in that number that we commonly buried four or five in a morning for the first four days.[1]

John Pringle, chief physician of the British Army at the Battle of Culloden in Scotland in 1746, showed that both soldiers and war prisoners in jail suffered the identical symptoms and that all of these fevers were a single entity. Its symptoms began with headache and a low fever, followed by a skin rash and delirium; stupor and death frequently ensued after two weeks. [2]

The Spread of Disease

A French naval squadron under the Duc D'Anville in Nova Scotia was afflicted with this fever and, upon departure for Europe, left behind some blankets and clothing in their encampment site. These were appropriated by a passing party of Mimack Indians, who took them back to their village. Almost the entire tribe succumbed to typhus. By the end of the eighteenth century, soiled clothing was looked upon with suspicion, and most naval surgeons took sanitary measures when the disease presented and sought to isolate infected crew members.[3]

Typhus broke out on the British vessel, *Juno,* carrying British marines and American prisoners of war, en route to Halifax, Nova Scotia, from New York in 1776. To overcome the disease, she was thoroughly scrubbed and disinfected. It is not known whether the crowded prisoners in the hold were part of this cleanup, but the disease was brought under control. She was then ordered to accept sixty supernumeraries from the accompanying *Rainbow,* eight of whom were febrile. The *Juno's* captain remonstrated with the fleet officer, and the febrile transfers were returned to the *Rainbow*—but too late. With a crew of about two hundred, plus the marines and American prisoners, the sick list climbed to 512 and sixteen deaths were recorded.

The perception of the cause of this illness by crewmembers, who were surrounded by their sick mates, often revealed a depth of understanding about the nature of this ailment that escaped the surgeons and officers. In one instance the surgeon who was caring for a typhus victim gave him medication and, upon returning for a follow-up visit the next day, was unable to locate his patient. His shipmates had washed his clothing, blankets, and hammock and transferred him to another area on the deck. Their excuse to the surgeon for this action was "because it was lousy."[4]

The Modern Perspective

If you, the reader, imagine yourself as surgeon aboard a vessel at this time, faced with such a contagion, could you avoid considering a connection between lice and this disease?

You are familiar with the ship's log, and you have seen this disease in all latitudes, in frigid and tropical climates, in stormy and placid seas. You have watched its dread symptoms develop in rain, fog, and sunshine, and you know that its course is not influenced by the barometer or wind direction.

As a surgeon, you know that "ship fever" occurs in association with dirty clothing and that impressed seamen picked up from the gutters of Liverpool have been known to spread the disease throughout a ship—usually, however, without infecting the officers. You know from experience that a gun crew transferred from a diseased ship to your healthy ship can infect most of the crew. As far as you know, when the disease is rampant, cleaning up the crew and disinfecting the ship controls the disease. On the other hand, you recall many previous voyages in which the crew wore filthy, unwashed clothes but no disease developed.

Your training at medical school taught you that the disease is caused by dirty clothes and toxic air emanating from a fouled environment, but this reasoning does not completely coincide with your experience on board. Once the disease has spread, getting rid of the foul air by opening ports and hatches has little effect. You know that the stricken crews were lice infested and showed the bites of lice on their bodies. But you discount this observation, because you know that the entire population, particularly the unbathed population, often carry lice and that this condition is ubiquitous on land as well as at sea. At this time no one had ever suggested or even considered an insect as a vector of any disease.

However, if you, as surgeon, have a scientific bent and are widely read, you will know about the discovery of a mite, genus *Acarus,* that can be seen under a magnifying lens, and that it is said to be responsible for scabies; so insects had been associated with disease![5] Unfortunately, you would know little or nothing of the scientific method of studying experimental and control groups, which was not well known or practiced at that time.

Would you, the reader, given the stated known and unknown facts of medical knowledge in the eighteenth century, have suspected lice to play a role in the transmission of typhus fever?

The prevailing theory of toxic air could so well explain the phenomenon of typhus fever, as well as all other bacterial and viral infections, that it was never challenged. Even now, wrongful theories certainly abound with which we feel psychologically comfortable and which we thus fail to question.

Controlling Typhus

By the end of the eighteenth century, soiled clothing was looked upon with suspicion and most naval surgeons isolated infected crew members and enforced sanitary measures. Bed-clothing and apparel were to be changed and washed weekly and aired on deck. Decks were washed with vinegar and walls whitewashed. The surgeon, however, was powerless to implement these measures unless he could convince the captain of their importance in maintaining the crew's ability to work..

In spite of fumigation, whitewashing, and so on, it was not uncommon for one or more ships to be completely withdrawn from service because of continued illness of the crew. James I sent his son Charles to Madrid to seek the hand of the Infanta and unite the two major seafaring nations by marriage. The newly built ship *Bonadventure* was to transport the happy couple back to England.

In a pathetic letter to the Lord Treasurer, Middlesex, the captain of the *Bonadventure,* Edward Christianson, requested that the ship be put out of service because of illness aboard. He wrote,

> I have not whereof to write but of the weake, and I may truely say Miserable
> estate of this Shippe. May your honour please to be assured that for one hun-

dred-sixty men, there is but seventy persons of all sortes that at present, is either fitt or able to do the Least Labour in the shippe of all the whole Company. When they are at the best, there is not twenty helme men, and but three that can heave a leade. I cannot Imagene how she came to be soe ill Manned. And the Inffection amongst us is most fearfull, sodarnely taken with amasedness and destraction whereof six are decayed and many at present as Mad as any in Bedlam—what corse to take. . . . I know not but to quit the ship of them as soone as possible.

In his reply, Middlesex wisely proposed not to add to the crew but to contain the disease. "His Majesty will perceive how grievouslie she is infected and therefore unfitt for such a passage . . . therefore the shippe shall come in and her men be discharged; and that the shippe may be clensed and made sweete and wholesome for future employment."[6]

Typhus can cause delirious behavior, so the reference to Bedlam points to the lice-borne scourge as the cause of the captain's distress. At it turned out, the engagement match never materialized, and the ship returned without a betrothed couple.

In another incident in 1739 an entire fleet was put out of commission by sickness. A large fleet of the Royal Navy was anchored off Spithead with the crews "so ill from the foul air of the ships" that the Admiralty ordered them ashore to recover their health. "The ships stank and infected one another." If a disagreeable odor was detected, it was thought to indicate disease, and the solution was to replace the odor with one that was freshly scented. The vessels were fumigated with smoke and washed down with hot vinegar. Ashore, the men bathed and laundered their bedding and clothes. Such widespread illness in people in close contact was usually in fact typhus.

In 1780 a most malignant fever was raging on board the *Edgar,* one of the largest ships in the fleet. Her surgeon, Mr. Robertson, informed Captain Elliott and recommended that the ship be removed from service and "to smoke the ship frequently with tobacco."

Robertson prescribed, "The tobacco ought to be well wet with vinegar and laid on fires placed in tubs, having water and shot under them." Two pounds of tobacco were placed over seven fires; all the ports and hatches were closed with tarpaulins.

Captain Elliott gave Robertson a free hand, and the *Edgar* was smoked five times; a little sulfur was mixed with the tobacco to prevent the men from appropriating it. A month later, Robertson reported only four fever patients. Lice succumb to high temperatures and smoke, and the general cleansing of the ship may also have helped. He suggested to Captain Elliott that he inform the Lords Commissioners of the Admiralty of the good effects of fumigation with tobacco, and Elliott did so. The surgeon of the *Prudent* also forwarded to the Admiralty his recommendation of the procedure. In neither case did their Lordships respond.[7]

Tropical Fevers

On anchoring a ship, the crew was again subject to disease. In tropical climates, intermittent or remittent fevers occurred, particularly if the anchorage was close to shore or an offshore breeze was blowing toxic air (in fact, mosquitoes) toward the ship. The men of some ships riding at anchor were fever-ridden while the crew of another ship, anchored one hundred yards away, remained healthy.

In tropical latitudes, crewmembers assigned to go ashore on watering details to fill the casks and cut firewood often developed fever. Such details, when forced to remain ashore for the night, greased their skin and huddled around fires to protect themselves from the toxic elements. James Lind did note that the sickening coastal air carried "moschitos," but there are no references or any comments in the literature of this period about mosquitoes as vectors of tropical diseases. Medical teaching was unanimous that the air was responsible for the fever, just as lice were overlooked as responsible for ship fever (typhus). In both instances the air quality was thought to be the cause of the disease.[8]

Lind recommended,

> I would advise all those who are cutting wood or in other laborious and dangerous services in hot climates during the heat of the day to have their heads covered with a bladder dipt in vinegar and to wash the mouth often with vinegar, never to swallow the spittle but rather to chew a little rhubarb. . . . to stop their nostrils with a small piece of linen or tow dipt in camphorated vinegar. . . . In the evening, leave off work. For their safety during the night on land, they should retire to a closed hut . . . a constant fire should be kept. . . . The smoking of tobacco . . . and chewing of garlic . . . are circumstances that will contribute to their preservation.

As a matter of fact, these measures, designed to limit as much contact as possible with toxic air, will also be somewhat effective against mosquitoes.[9]

John Hunter

John Hunter, outstanding surgeon, teacher, and researcher, when stationed in Jamaica as army surgeon, wrote that one-third of the force was sick at all times in this outpost. He noted that air near the marshy coast was very pernicious and the men were often febrile, while those troops at higher levels were healthy. He reported that, in a period of four years, 3,500 men died with fever, so that constant troop replacements were necessary.

Hunter wrote to the War Department in London, urging the rebuilding of the coastal barracks on a point of high land and, knowing the concerns of the administration, cleverly argued that such a move would reduce the logistical expense of constant troop replacement. He knew that a humanitarian argument, dependent on health issues and the salvage of the lives of the soldiers, would carry little weight. In any event, the war department took no action on his plea.

Hunter studied the fevers in his Jamaican post and sorted them into two types. Remittent fever (possibly yellow fever) caused chills with high temperatures, headaches, vomiting, and weakness, and it remitted with no regularity; it was often associated with yellow skin and eyes and frequently resulted in early death. Intermittent fever (malaria) recurred at regular intervals and responded to cinchona tree bark (quinine).[10]

William Baldwin

Whampoa in China, on the other side of the world from Jamaica, is a large seaport near Canton that was an important port of entry for American and European merchant vessels in the eighteenth century. In July 1807, twenty American merchant vessels rode at anchor in the harbor. William Baldwin, a recent medical graduate, was surgeon on the *New Jersey*, 125 days out of Philadelphia.

The crew was in excellent health during the long voyage but suffered illness soon after anchoring. Baldwin attributed the ill health of the crew to the low marshy ground bordering the harbor, which flooded with each high tide. The weather was sultry, the temperatures between 80 and 90 degrees Fahrenheit, with frequent thundershowers. All the American crews were confined to the harbor area for several months, while the captains and agents traveled to nearby cities and purchased cargo for the return journey to America. Meanwhile, Baldwin was treating remittent fever and dysentery due, he thought, to the morbid exhalations of the harbor and the stench of the swamp miasmas circulating throughout the area. He believed that the change of food, exposure to the hot sun, and sleeping on the damp deck at night were contributing causes.

The mainstay of his treatment was bleeding, which Hunter, in a similar situation in Jamaica, had found useless. Nevertheless, Baldwin stated, "This evacuation was always attended with the happiest effect, affording an almost immediate mitigation of the most alarming and distressing symptoms."

Baldwin's teaching was influenced by Benjamin Rush of Philadelphia. Rush vigorously denied that there was more than one disease suffered by humankind. All symptoms were different stages of one disease, so a single therapy sufficed for all maladies. The most effective treatment advocated by Rush was bleeding.

The experience of Baldwin, who believed bleeding cured his crew of "the fevers," demonstrates the hazards of interpreting anecdotal evidence about what is effective and what is not, in a disease whose course is self-limited or recurrent. Symptoms might subside even if no treatment were given.[11] Hunter at least recognized the differences between diseases, although he had no knowledge of the causes or any specific therapy for such diseases.

John Milne

John Milne spent five years as surgeon on two voyages to Whampoa, China, from London (1793–98) on the *Carnatic* and the *Dublin*. His crew also arrived in Whampoa in good health. As an experienced surgeon, he persuaded his captains to send the gunner with a water detail of natives to fill the casks from streams high in the mountains, far removed from the polluted waters of the harbor area. He reported no fevers in Whampoa, and his crew remained in good health during their stay. Milne avoided the dysenteries that plagued Baldwin, but both had cases of malaria. Milne may have depended on quinine rather than bleeding, which suppressed malaria, but we have no record of his having done so.[12]

Chapter 7

Death and Disease in the Slave Trade

THE SOCIAL ILLS concurrent with the age of sail further burdened sea surgeons, who had to treat the consequences of hazardous work, deadly warfare, and brutal punishments, as well as dietary and infectious diseases, in ships' crews. To this was added the paramount social ill, the slave trade, and its attendant maladies.

In the fifteenth century, when the first slave traders sailed into the bays of West Africa and followed the river paths into the interior, the economic, cultural, and political structure of this area changed forever.

Before their arrival, peaceful and stable agricultural communities, ruled by tribal chiefs, traded with each other. The inhabitants were described as friendly, intelligent, and industrious. Occasionally, there had been contacts with European traders who sailed up the rivers and lived among the tribes in a friendly relationship. The people were hospitable and visitors welcomed and protected; it was a capital offense to injure a foreigner.[1] Then came the slave trade.

A contemporary of Captain Hawkins, an English sea captain and explorer, reported that in 1562 the captain purchased a boatload of slaves at the mouth of the Nunez River in Sierra Leone.[2] Hawkins opened traffic to English vessels that would trade in slaves from West African ports for more than two hundred years. His original human cargo was sold in Hispaniola in exchange for hides, sugar, and other New World products, but he had only a passing interest in the slave trade. His main interest was exploration, and his voyages to distant lands in a long seafaring career were widely read. Late in his life, Queen Elizabeth recognized his explorations and knighted him.[3]

By 1618 the slave trade was established as a profitable commercial enterprise pursued by vessels from England, France, Spain, and Portugal.

James I of England granted a charter to Sir Albert Rich to establish a company for the purpose of collecting and shipping slaves from West Africa. Another company, chartered in 1662, agreed to supply three thousand slaves annually to Jamaica, but we have no record of whether it filled its quota or how long it continued to operate.

The West African coast and inland as far as five hundred miles was the setting for this trade. On the Horn of Africa on the northeastern and eastern coasts, Arabian traders had carried on a slave market even before this period, but it never reached the magnitude of the operations on the west coast. A medical dimension soon became apparent in this commerce. European traders following the river routes of West Africa risked sickness and death from dysentery, guinea worms, yaws, craw-craw (scabies), elephantiasis, and sleeping sickness.[4]

The abolitionist Falconbridge published *An Account of the Slave Trade on the Coast of Africa* in 1788. In it he describes slavery-as-usual in vivid detail. Sometimes fifteen or more ships lay at the mouth of the Bonny River in Sierra Leone while other vessels combed the coast, each captain intent on purchasing several hundred slaves. As demand rose in the New World, the slavers used elaborate strategies to increase the supply of slaves. Tribal kings along the coast were enticed to become brokers and provide ship captains with cargoes of slaves. Competing captains wined and dined them and offered them extravagant gifts in exchange for their help.

In a typical slaving negotiation, a ship, upon entering a harbor and anchoring, would send a message to the local king, inviting him and his party on board for dinner. As the royal boat approached the vessel, a blast from a horn made of an hollow elephant tusk would announce its arrival. And, as the Africans came aboard, they would see the items for trade displayed on the trader's deck: cotton, silk, brandy, firearms, and cutlasses.[5] When the king and his retinue returned to shore, the ship would fire a salute in his honor.[6] The crew then prepared the ship for the arrival of the slaves.

Collecting a complete slave cargo could take several months, during which time many slaves had to be housed aboard ship before the transatlantic journey began. A few slaves would be gathered at every port, and the vessel made multiple anchorages at different ports along the coast. The crew had rigged a ridge pole and supports on deck, forming a structure covered with rushes, and the deck surface was extended about two feet on either side to increase the holding area. A partition in the enclosure separated the sexes, and the edges of the enclosure were reinforced so that none could escape by jumping overboard. Peepholes in the enclosure were made for muskets in case of insurrection. An enclosure of this kind protected those in the corral from the direct rays of the tropical sun but not from heavy rain showers, and the heat was stifling inside.[7] When the ship began the transatlantic crossing, the victims were removed from the deck and herded below into the hold, chained in pairs.

* * *

Typically, two or three slaves were boarded daily, occasionally more. If a shortage loomed, the native brokers fomented wars between previously peaceful tribes, promising the aggressor king booty for captured prisoners. If the king protested and refused to cooperate, mysterious fires erupted during the night and entire villages were torched. Probably, more people were killed, injured, and made homeless in these forays than the number of prisoners secured. Kidnapping was another method used to satisfy the increasing demand.

Now the ship was ready to receive its human cargo. If there were many competing vessels in the harbor, the prices went up.

Ship surgeons were required to examine the purchased slaves before they were boarded, eliminating those with wounds or diseases and those otherwise incapable of hard labor. When surgeons reported that they saw few wounded, it was assumed that most of the slaves in the barricaded holding compound on shore had been kidnapped. Gangs roamed the countryside, kidnapping solitary workers in the fields, and raided villages at night, collecting those people who were acceptable as slaves and killing the rest. Raiders then battled each other for their human booty, until the social structure crumbled and anarchy and fear swept over threatened areas.

Falconbridge describes an incident in which a young man was invited by a slave broker to his house for a meal and, upon leaving, was treacherously seized; struggling, he escaped, but was chased and set upon by a large dog kept for that purpose and recaptured. Children assigned by their parents to scare off the birds in a newly seeded field were especially vulnerable to kidnapping. Another incident related by Falconbridge was that of a friend invited by his neighbor to take him close to a vessel to view it. He agreed, trusting his neighbor, and was rowed alongside a ship where he was overcome by several native traders and sold. Even the kidnappers were kidnapped.

The judicial system was not immune to the taint of foreign money and became totally corrupt. Those tried and convicted by a native court for minor offenses were sold to brokers. Courts became so venal that people were tried on trumped-up charges, convicted, and sold. Interrogation of prisoners by the ship surgeons who were examining them revealed that ultimately more prisoners were being fed into the hands of the brokers by kidnappers, raiders, and the court system than by tribal warfare. If by chance a wealthy or important person was captured, his friends were contacted and instructed to pay a ransom for his release.

When the coastal areas were depleted of victims, the brokers turned inland, following the river system for additional captives who were collected, tied together, and marched to the distant coast, herded by guards armed with muskets. When asked how long they had been marching, they replied, "several moons." One observer estimated that of every twelve captives that began the march, only seven survived to reach the coast.[8]

When a large number of prisoners was thus collected on the coast, rather than taking them aboard immediately, the brokers put them in detention pens.[9] The old, infirm, and sick who had survived the march were weeded out and reportedly killed by drowning. Lameness, narrow chests, deformities, bad eyes, or bad teeth were causes for rejection. In the detention pens, after the weeding-out procedure, the remaining slaves were cleaned and their skins oiled with palm oil so that they would look healthier and bring a better price.

When a captain agreed to a purchase from the detention pen, he sent his surgeon to select the most healthy bodies. Once they were loaded on board, the captain and the surgeon did a second examination and the unfit were rowed back to shore—screaming, as they knew that a return to shore as unwanted merchandise was to be put to death.

While brokers scoured the interior for captives, areas of the coast where ships had not been trading for several years returned to a peaceful way of life. On the coast of Angola, at the mouth of the river Ambris, no slaver had appeared for several years and the tribes had resumed their peaceful coexistence, when a ship arrived. Brokers renewed warfare that brought them many prisoners for sale.

Finally, in 1788, Parliament, under pressure from the abolitionists, passed a law regulating British ships in the slave trade. It was estimated that prior to that year 150,000 were taken from the west coast of Africa

annually. After 1788, the slave trade continued unabated by the Portuguese, French, and Spanish but was limited in British ships. Entrenched
British slave-ship owners defeated a series of abolitionist proposals in Parliament, but a law was finally passed in 1807 prohibiting any British ship
from transporting slaves. British slave trading continued illegally, until it
was finally suppressed by warships patrolling the collection areas in West
Africa.

On 22 March 1794, the United States Congress passed a bill signed by
President Washington prohibiting the transportation of slaves from the
United States to any foreign country, but it did not interfere with the continued transportation of slaves from Africa to the United States. Article I,
section 9, of the United States Constitution stated that after 1808 the
power of the states to control immigration and the passage of individuals
into states was to be regulated by Congress. While the power of immigration still resided within the states, by 1800 every state but South Carolina
made importation of slaves illegal, although enforcement of the laws
remained lax.

The abolitionist movement in Britain had been gaining momentum
since the early eighteenth century, and abolitionists were increasingly
active in Africa. A letter from the British governor of Sierra Leone, dated
3 August 1709, angrily condemned the abolitionists who were infiltrating
his colony as "hypocrites" seeking to destroy the slave trade. He accused
them of a conspiracy to provide cheap labor for their farms in Africa. He
also accused them of instilling ideas of liberty in the black community
and fomenting a lack of respect for government and the courts. As a
result, he charged that crime had increased and the streets were unsafe.
The letter's ranting, illogical tone was doubtless due to his anger at being
called back to London to answer for his conduct in obstructing the
abolitionists.[10]

In the United States, an 1806 federal law prohibiting importation of
slaves was not seriously enforced until 1820.

Practicing Medicine on Slave Ships

Most accounts of African culture and the collection of slaves that are
available for study were written by authors with strong abolitionist lean-
ings, and some exaggeration and worst-case scenarios may be expected
from an aggressive group seeking to convince others of the inhumanity of

slavery. The general truth of these reports would seem to be recorded faithfully, but some magnification of numbers and selection of unusual events and reports were possible.

Falconbridge, a determined abolitionist, repeatedly described the number of slaves transported in a single ship to be between six and seven hundred.[11] An anonymous author also stated that six to seven hundred were sometimes loaded on board.[12] Winterbottom quoted a surgeon by the name of Phillips who stated that his ship carried seven hundred slaves in a voyage from Guinea to the Barbados, of whom 320 died of various diseases.[13]

Ships made the round-trip journey in three passages. The first passage was between Liverpool, Bristol, Hull, London, or other British ports to Sierra Leone or other landings on the west coast of Africa, carrying cloth, firearms, liquor, or manufactured goods for trading. The second passage was between Africa and the Caribbean or North or South America, with cargoes of slaves. The third passage was a return to England with sugar, rum, or cotton.

The number of slaves transported and the deaths quoted by the abolitionists can be compared with the manifest reports and the logs of surgeons of various ships in the trade, which record both the numbers transported in each ship and the mortality to be much less than given in the literature. The surgeon's figures were certified by officers of the ports to which the slaves were delivered. Several surgeons' records of the transportation of these wretched cargoes were available for study.

Between October 1788 and 31 March 1789 Dr. David Jones was surgeon on the slave ship *Friendship* en route from London to the Cape Coast in Africa and from there to Lucea, Jamaica, where the ship registered at customs. Jones recorded the names and illnesses of crewmembers, who were diagnosed as having intermittent fever (malaria or yellow fever), bilious fever (hepatitis or other diseases), and dysentery. The specific illnesses of the slaves were not diagnosed or recorded, but they were listed as sick or recovered and the surgeon's visits to them were also recorded. Jones proudly asserts that he had had no deaths amongst the slaves or crew since their departure from London. He listed twenty-five slaves aboard, which is an unusually small number.[14]

The surgeon's report from the ship *Ned* described the dates and numbers of slaves collected each day while anchored off the coast of Guinea between 17 November and 20 December 1788. Two hundred and seventy-nine slaves were boarded, and by the ship's arrival in the West Indies, twenty-five had died. The diseases afflicting the slaves were listed in the log to include bilious fever, insanity, lethargy, decline, and one fatal case of gangrene of the leg. The last could have been caused by damage to the tissues from a leg iron.

Dr. James Watts, surgeon of the *Mary*, recorded that she was anchored off the west coast of Africa between 16 July 1788 and 13 February 1789, seeking cargo. It took seven months to collect two hundred slaves before she set sail for the West Indies on the middle passage. She arrived at Roseau in Dominica, where the surgeon certified to the port authority that three slaves had died. One died of gangrene of the leg, again probably from a leg-iron injury; the second died of "anasarca and hydrocele" (generalized swelling and perhaps beriberi or heart or kidney disease); the third died of "swelling of the knee," most likely sepsis from an infection of the knee joint.

James Buckham was surgeon on board the *James* from November 1788 to February 1789. The total number of slaves carried was 154 and fourteen deaths were recorded, ten from dysentery, the remaining from "inflammation of the liver, lethargy and sulkiness." One crewmember died of pleurisy on this voyage.

The ship *Lively*, Joseph Hinchcliffe, surgeon, cruised the African west coast from September through October of 1788; on some days she loaded as many as forty-two slaves, on other days only one or two. The surgeon reported that any slaves in the detention camp who were ill were left there until recovered; if a boarded slave became ill, he was returned to shore. After 374 slaves were collected, the *Lively* began her transatlantic crossing, arriving in Roseau, Dominica, after a voyage of six weeks, having lost thirteen en route. The diagnoses given as the cause of death included quinsy, "decline," palsy, measles, insanity, and complaints in the bowels. Even in the eighteenth century many of these were not acceptable diagnoses as a cause of death.

The *Madame Pookate*, with Benjamin Smith, surgeon, aboard, collected 183 slaves, and his log yields some information about ages and sex as well as numbers. It carried "forty-seven men, twenty-two women (eight women with children feeding at the breast), twenty-four boys over four feet, four inches in height, forty-four boys under this height, twelve girls over four feet, four inches, and twenty-six girls under this height." Six died during the voyage, and the surgeon's log gave as the causes of death "inflammation, apoplexy, bilious fever, flux [dysentery]."

A more complete account of the medical problems on board a slave ship was recorded by Christopher Bowen, surgeon of the *Lord Stanley*, which was cruising the African coast between 23 March and 25 June 1792. The hold was filled with 389 people, who were divided by age and sex as follows: 214 men, 67 man-boys, 10 boys, 68 women, 24 women-girls, and 6 girls. Bowen kept a detailed log of the ill patients and their progress, giving each sick person a number and describing the patient's symptoms, treatment, and progress. On his rounds, below deck in the hold, he saw approximately eight patients a day, and most recovered. Before setting sail, he returned to the shore several who were lame and one epileptic. Seventeen died during the crossing, almost all of these with dysentery, but many others suffered from diarrhea and recovered.

The *Lord Stanley* passed customs on the fourteenth of August in St. George, Grenada.[15]

This diary was later reviewed by Dr. Ronald Ross of the Liverpool School of Tropical Medicine in 1911, who suggested that many of the illnesses and the deaths could be accounted for by a syndrome similar to infantile diarrhea, but he also suggested that self-inflicted poisoning must be considered. Such conclusions are unacceptable in the light of present-day knowledge, and it is much more likely that the illnesses and deaths were from infectious dysenteries and typhoid, with resulting dehydration and bowel complications.

The figures for the number of slaves transported in these ships and the deaths during transport were supplied by the various surgeons and certified under oath to the customs officers at the debarkation points. The average number carried per ship was 201 slaves. If we remove the figures from the ship carrying only twenty-five as an outlier, the average number carried increases to 238. The average number of deaths during the crossing was 7 or 3 percent. These figures are far different from those quoted by the abolitionists, who used their figures to pressure Parliament to pass additional reform legislation. On the other hand, these figures were all from the period of 1788 or later, when restrictive legislation was already on the books, and it was mandatory for the surgeon to forward his reports to London.

These figures invite comparison with those of the crowded convict ships transporting criminals from England to New South Wales, Australia. The first convict fleet in 1798 had few casualties because Surgeon

Bowes maintained strict cleanliness, frequent airing of the ships, and exercise for the prisoners. The second fleet in 1790 recorded death and disease similar to the slave ships on their transatlantic crossings. There were 226 women convicts on the *Lady Juliana* and about four hundred men transported on the *Neptune*. Disease was particularly recorded on the *Neptune*, which was carrying the men, of whom 171 died. They were chained below decks for the entire voyage for a year, never exercised, and given reduced rations.

Joseph Smith, aged sixteen, was described in Flynn's history as "chained below in the darkness with light from a few oil lamps occasionally lighted." The chains clinked and rattled as the ship rolled and pitched. Saltwater washed down the hatches in heavy seas, and the stench was ever present, accompanied by the coughing and the groans of the dying. He suffered from constant hunger and the pain of leg sores from the irons. He tried not to think of his hunger as he grew thinner and weak; sometimes a kind crewmember would slip him a piece of bread or cheese, once even a lump of sugar, which he fondly remembered for days. On the other hand the *Lady Juliana*, which carried the women, did not chain the convicts and allowed them freedom of the deck, and few deaths were recorded. The captain of the *Neptune* and the victualler were later tried in court in London and convicted of malfeasance and inhumanity.[16]

Comparing the deaths of the male convicts on the *Neptune* and the slaves on the slave ships, it would appear that the number carried was less important than the conditions in which they were transported. Chaining the convicts and slaves led to filth and total absence of hygiene and, along with the lack of exercise and poor food, caused a high mortality. It was the captain who was responsible for these conditions, and the record affirms that slave-ship captains were unscrupulous. The few deaths on the *Lady Juliana* underscore these conclusions. Convict and slave ships had in common the poor food, the lack of exercise, the filth, and the chaining in the hold.

The slave trade, with its attendant human misery and the large fortunes that could be quickly amassed, attracted avaricious captains who had little regard for life. They were looked down upon by other members of their profession, and their inhuman behavior was directed not only to their human cargo but to their officers, crews, and surgeons. Many atrocities directed toward the crew were recorded in this period. In one, an elderly sailor who complained about the water was beaten and forced to swallow a pump bolt.[17]

The more slaves delivered, the greater was the captain's profit, which was shared with the owner of the vessel in Liverpool, Bristol, or another coastal city in Europe. Discipline was cruelly administered on these ships, and the mortality of seamen higher than on others. Not only slaves sought to escape this environment. Winterbottom on more than one occasion witnessed crewmembers, chiefs, and second mates, as well as surgeons, desert the stifling command of a venal captain and take refuge in the colony at Sierra Leone.[18]

On leaving England, most ships engaged in the African trade carried a crew of thirty to forty. The number on the ship's return to England on the third passage, ten to eighteen months after leaving, was about half that, because of death, illness, and desertions.[19] The crews of these ships were drawn from the lowest social orders and included drunkards, criminals, and those indebted to a public ale house who were delivered to the captains under threat of being thrown into debtor's prison.

The food was poor and often spoiled in the warm climate, while tropical diseases took their toll. The voyages were dangerous because of slave revolts, mutinies, and criminal activities on board, as well as pirate raids and the usual tropical storms and hurricanes. Captains did not strive to improve the crew's conditions; after all, a dead or deserted seaman was one less mouth to feed on the return journey, on which fewer crew were necessary.

More often than not, the surgeons on these ships were recent graduates of medical school, usually poor, without other opportunities to practice. Once lured into the slave trade by necessity, they found that their sensibilities were offended and frequently their health ruined. Most surgeons completed a single trip and did not re-enlist.

A sea surgeon was in continual conflict with the captain. If he refused to pass a slave who appeared to be in ill health, he was overruled by the captain. If that slave died en route, the surgeon was blamed for the death. His recommendations for exercise, food, and medications for the slaves were refused, yet when a slave died the surgeon was held personally responsible.[20]

Thomas Trotter, as a young doctor recently discharged from the Royal Navy and seeking work, enlisted as a surgeon on a slaver. In his later life he became fleet surgeon to the Channel Fleet and personal physician to Admiral Lord Howe, and on retirement he became a writer, poet, and reformer. He described his experiences on the Guineaman *Brooks*, scouring the coast of Africa for slaves between July and the following March before the quota of one hundred slaves was collected.

In his firsthand account of his voyage, Trotter wrote about the plight of the slaves chained below deck and unable to move freely, growing fat from a diet of beans, corn, rice, and guinea pepper. After several months of cruising the coast, he noted early signs of scurvy. Trotter argued with the captain to permit them on deck daily for exercise when the weather would permit, at which time the hold could be cleaned and aired. He noted that the slaves liked to dance to the tune of drums, and this could be encouraged on deck, but on Trotter's vessel the captain refused his pleas. Allowing the slaves on deck and unshackling them provided an opportunity to escape, and profits might be reduced.

When they were allowed on deck, to prevent insurrection a long chain bolted to a deck plate at both ends was passed through the leg irons of the slaves. Those who were regarded as dangerous were also secured to the ship by neck irons.[21]

Olaudah Equiano

Olaudah Equiano, an eleven-year-old child, was playing with his friends in a remote village near Sierra Leone when he was kidnapped by a band of black slavers and marched to the coast, where he was loaded on a slave ship bound for the island of Barbados. Equiano became a personal servant to a captain of the Royal Navy, fought in naval battles, and traveled widely. When in England, he was sent to school and learned to read, and he wrote a book about his experiences, *The Interesting Narrative of Olaudah Equiano or Gustavus Vassa,* published in 1789. ("Gustavus Vassa" was the name given him by his master.) Later he was freed and traveled throughout England, lecturing against the ancient and persisting evils of slavery in the abolitionist cause.

His account of his voyage aboard the slave ship shows us firsthand the agony of those chained in the hold. He was bundled aboard the ship by his black captors, shivering with fear and convinced that those red-faced men with long hair who spoke a language he had never heard were about to eat him. His kidnappers tried to calm him, speaking his native language, but they soon received their money and left. He was offered food by the white men and beaten when he refused to eat it. He was sent below to experience "a loathsome stench such as I had never experienced."

At first he was chained in the hold, but because of his youth he was sometimes permitted on deck. The surgeon would request that those mortally ill be allowed on deck to escape the foul air below, and Olaudah watched as two of these captives, chained together, threw themselves overboard. The ship hove to and the boat lowered, but one was drowned, and the survivor returned to be brutally flogged. Equiano frequently considered escaping by jumping into the ocean.

Chained below, he was so crowded he had no room to turn around. Above the shrieks of the women and the groans of the dying, he recognized his language somewhere distant in the hold and found familiar faces from his village. What was going to happen to him? Where was he going? They told him he was bound for a new land, where he would work for the white people, but he was not reassured. He was still convinced that he would be killed, "for I have never seen among my people such instances of brutal cruelty, and this was not only shown towards us blacks, but also to some of the whites themselves."[22]

In spite of the filth and inhumane surroundings, friendships among the slaves were forged, made in the darkness of the hold during the long weeks of the voyage. Their common destiny—their experiences and origins in Africa and their forced voyage to a new land—bound them in a brotherhood that endured for a lifetime.

The women and girls were kept in a separate hold and were not chained, and the captains turned a blind eye to crewmembers who bribed or cajoled them for their favors.

Food consisted of beans boiled to a pulp with boiled yams and rice and a small quantity of pork or beef (often skimmed from the rations of the crew), provided twice daily, and a daily allowance of one half-pint of water. Several buckets were placed in each hold for stools and urine and emptied once daily. To use them, the person desiring to relieve himself had to drag his chained partner in the darkness of the hold, stumbling and falling over bodies on the floor, their chains entangling, with resulting anger, curses, and fights, before an overfilled bucket could be reached. Soon efforts to reach a bucket were abandoned, and the deck itself became a receptacle.

Slaves were much more prone to seasickness than the working crew, and their vomit added to the foul-smelling, slimy mixture coating the deck. Indeed, it is surprising that sickness was not more prevalent and that epidemics of bacillary and amoebic dysentery, hepatitis, scurvy, measles, smallpox, and cholera did not decimate the holds. Typhus was not reported by any of its common names, possibly because there was no bedding used and almost no clothing was worn that could harbor the lice.

The diseases among the slaves that were recorded in the surgeons' reports to the House of Lords were dysentery or flux, injuries from chains, and abdominal complaints. To the surgeon attending the sick in these circumstances, it was insufferable work, and he could not remain below longer than fifteen minutes.[23] Yet most surgeons visited the sick daily, made notes in their journals, and recorded their patient's progress.

It was also the responsibility of the surgeon to inspect the water and food supply and to make certain that each person received a fair share. After the law restricting slave transport was passed by Parliament, it was also the responsibility of the surgeon to testify about the health and treatment of slaves on board. After passing customs, it was common for the captain to send the sick slaves ashore under guard, along with the surgeon charged with restoring their health. One surgeon describes being sent ashore with one hundred slaves and being housed with them in an old building for twelve days. Some died and most did not improve in this time.

Mutiny and Uprising

With the amalgam of personalities thrown together on these crossings, including the profiteering captains, the criminal element in the crew, and prisoner slaves, it is not unexpected that mutinies, insurrections, and violence would ignite. Slave suicide attempts were common. In the detention camps, eating soil resulted in skin pallor, puffy eyes, and weakness but seldom had the desired effect of death. A more effective way to commit suicide was drowning after jumping overboard whenever an opportunity was offered. Sometimes slaves escaped their bonds on board, and rebellion, chaos, and bloodshed followed.

John Harris, a crewmember of the Guineaman *Marlborough,* wrote a firsthand report to his father that was published in Bristol on 24 March 1753.

Hon Father   Bonney Oct 25, 1752

This is to let you know what a bad Misfortune I have met with—The 11th of this Instant we got over the bar at Bonney and the 14th following, being a fine Day our Captain thought proper to wash the slaves, so orderd Tubs and Swabs to be got ready, all the People being busy except the Centries: The Gold Coast slaves rose upon the quarter deck and alarmed the whole ship, knocked the Centries down at the Barricade and tossed them overboard.

The slaves then armed themselves and attacked the captain who escaped by scrambling up the ratlines to the fore top. The remaining crew had no weapons and armed themselves with staves. The boatswain's mate and other crew members were killed. What crew remained fled up the rigging while the slaves fired at them from below. The surgeon and some crew members got into the punt trying to escape and were shot and clubbed. Perceiving the surgeon was not dead they got the cook's Mall and beat his brains out.

The chief mate was then stabbed, the second mate had his throat slit "from ear-to-ear." The third mate in the rigging was shot and made his way to the deck pleading for mercy, but was cut from limb to limb.

[Harris, the writer, was shot in the belly and in the arm, but was able to hang onto the rigging.]

A few hours later, seeing only a few of the crew was left, the slaves let them come down from the rigging—all except the captain. They singled out the author of the letter, calling his name, shoved him along the deck and chained him to the cabin. When the slaves found out there were still twelve crew left, they decided to reduce this number, and threw four overboard.

The remaining were ordered to put the ship about and start for the land, which they reached in two days.

At this time an intertribal dispute developed between the Gold Coast slaves and those from the Bonney area, when they overloaded the long boat in a frantic attempt to reach shore; they fought with each other for space in the longboat and many drowned.

They then cut the cable and the *Marlborough* drifted seaward, with eight crew still on board, and was lost.[24]

Violence of a different type erupted on the *Clayton* of Liverpool. On the night of 19 September 1752, she dropped anchor off the coast of Pernambuco, Brazil. Her mate slipped ashore unobserved during the night. He had been a prisoner aboard the *Clayton* and had just eluded his captors. He told the port authorities that while off the coast of Guinea in February 1752, nine British sailors of the crew robbed a neighboring ship anchored alongside. The renegades then returned to the *Clayton,* which was loaded with slaves and ready to depart. They fomented a mutiny of the crew, joined by about half of them, with the intention of crossing to South America to sell the slaves and pocket the money for themselves. We are not told what happened to the rest of the crew, but the captain was shot and set adrift in a small boat, and the mate made a prisoner and forced to navigate the mutineers to Brazil rather than the West Indies, the intended delivery port. On this passage, a large number of neglected slaves, without medical attention, died. Of the 450 that were loaded in Africa, 124 died. "Smallpox and other distempers" were given as the causes of death.

The mutinous crew was imprisoned by the Portuguese authorities, who auctioned the slaves; the proceeds of the sale were kept by Portugal and used to refit the vessel, and the excess appropriated by the King of Portugal. The ship then joined a convoy of eighteen merchant vessels escorted by a man-of-war with the imprisoned mutineers and docked at Lisbon. The owners of the ship petitioned the British secretary of state, William Pitt, describing the mutiny and requesting the money for the "sale of the goods." Presumably the ship was returned.[25]

On the *Marlborough* the slaves rose up and made an escape attempt that was partially successful but succumbed to intertribal feuding, with bloodshed on both sides. In the *Clayton*, they were witnesses to the avarice and criminal behavior of their captors, and silently and helplessly suffered.

Another famous rebellion of slaves occurred in July 1839, this time in Caribbean waters. Don Jose Ruiz and Don Pedro Montez of Cuba purchased fifty-three slaves recently arrived from Africa and put them on board the *Amistad*, Captain Ferrer commanding, in order to transport them to Principe in western Cuba. Four days out of Havana, the Africans armed themselves with sugarcane knives and attacked the captain and crew. Captain Ferrer and the cook were killed. Two of the crew escaped, and Ruiz and Montez were made prisoner. They escaped with their lives but lost a legal battle in the United States for ownership of the rebels.[26]

A more heartening story is the freeing of slaves and the confiscation of a slaver. In April 1823, after Britain had outlawed slave transport, slave runners from France, Spain, and Portugal were still collecting slaves in waters around the Bonney River, claimed by the British. A Royal Navy sloop was ordered to sail up the river to seek out any slave ships. Lieutenant Mildmay, in command, discovered the *Vigilante*, a French ship of two hundred tons, and three Spanish ships loading slaves. There were already 345 slaves on board when the battle erupted. In the commotion many jumped overboard and were attacked by sharks, but most were saved. On boarding the *Vigilante*, Mildmay discovered a twelve-year-old girl in a neck iron dragging a ten-foot length of chain, which he removed and placed on the captain of the *Vigilante*.[27]

* * *

The ravages inflicted on the communities of West Africa between the six-teenth and the nineteenth centuries have left their mark to this day. Health practices and efforts of physicians were of little avail to reduce the toll of death and disease under such conditions created by men without conscience.

Chapter 8

Impressment and Punishment

THE POPULATION of England had grown from five million during the reign of Queen Elizabeth to twelve million by the end of the eighteenth century. Royal Navy forces had increased to over 120,000 men. Moreover, larger ships were being built that required larger crews; for example, the *Edgar*, built in 1798, carried a crew of two thousand men.[1] A large annual infusion of manpower was needed to maintain the fleet.

But each year about five thousand crewmen died of disease. There always were some so ill that they could be of no service. In addition, the navy lost personnel by desertion; a sailor's was a harsh and dangerous life. Attrition was such that the pool of men available was never adequate, and the navy required more men each year. What was to be done?

Impressment

The impressment of seamen was a last resort for the Admiralty. Having tempted young men to join by offering bounties, and having been unsuccessful in this, the Admiralty tried a quota system whereby each county was compelled to provide a fixed number of seamen each year, but this was also ineffective. One answer to the problem was to take personnel by force.

The solution brought with it a hailstorm of other problems. Impressment into the navy of tramps and vagabonds in their filthy and verminous clothing and criminals from jail increased the incidence of disease, which spread to the volunteer yeomen. The impressed men were poor sailors, not only debilitated by malnutrition and disease but also likely to desert whenever an opportunity was available.

Near the Thames estuary, naval vessels lay in wait for unsuspecting merchantmen or colliers from Newcastle and, without warrants, sent marines on board and seized able-bodied sailors and transferred them to naval vessels. Once on board, the impressed men were urged to voluntarily sign on as crew and were offered inducements to do so. If they refused to sign, they were singled out for the most difficult and dangerous duties and given no leave.[2]

Impressment of seamen by the British Navy was an evil feared and hated by the general populace, but especially by sailors on leave, home from a voyage of many months, who would be kidnapped and forced aboard a navy ship ready to set sail to distant seas. Other young able-bodied men, living in seaport towns, who might be unemployed also faced this danger. On the seas, merchant vessels of all nations faced the danger of being overtaken by a warship and some of the crew forcibly removed.

Punishment

Sailors in this period endured severe privations that few mortals would accept. When the day-to-day life is so miserable, punishment, to be effective, has to be even more miserable. The power to flog served such a purpose, and when the captain or his officers were sadistic and lacked the imagination to inspire the crew by leadership, the lash was the answer.

John Wetherill, a seaman, described in his diary in 1803 the case of Henry Wilson, a seventeen-year-old boy, dragged out of a Harwich smack and impressed in the HMS *Hussar*. During the night the boy sought to return to his mother by jumping overboard and swimming to shore. He was soon found and returned to the *Hussar,* where he was put in leg irons awaiting the sentence of the captain for desertion.

> On the following morning he was brought forth to suffer from attempting to gain his liberty. . . . All hands were called . . . and marines all placed in the gangways and in front of the quarter deck, all under arms to protect the officers. The ship's master at arms reported the prisoner ready for punishment.
>
> From the quarter deck, the command came, "Seize him up, and as for you Boatswains mate, do your duty, or I will see your back bones."
>
> The boy pleaded, "Oh Captain for the sake of my mother, have mercy on me and forgive me."
>
> "No, sir, if I forgave you, I hope God will never forgive me. Go on, Boatswains mate."
>
> "Master-at-arms how many has he had?"
>
> "One dozen and five, Sir."
>
> The Captain replied, "Go on."

The boy fainted and lay as dead and the Captain accused him of play acting and repeated, "Go on."

The crew began to murmur and grow restless and if not for the marines might have stormed the quarter deck. After two dozen lashes, no signs of life were to be seen in the victim.

The surgeon, who had the power to terminate the punishment, felt the pulse of the victim and ordered the flogging to be ended. The captain was still not satisfied and said, "Your order shall be obeyed in that respect, but mine shall in another."

The boy was made fast with a rope and heaved overboard three times without showing any signs of life. Doctor Graham ordered him below and wrapped him in blankets. Later, he bled him as the lad began to groan and cry for his mother.[3]

Discipline and morale suffered as a result of impressment, making it necessary to mete out inhumane punishments that further discouraged volunteering. A parson visiting a ship described a seaman pinioned to the main mast, arms stretched out, with a marlin spike thrust into his mouth and held there for one hour while blood from his lacerated mouth ran down his chin. The offense was swearing.

Other punishments included ducking at the main yardarm, hauling the offender on a tackle high above the sea, and then dropping him into the surf. For more severe offenses, the punishment might be keelhauling. The seaman was dragged under the keel from one side to the other, his body tied to ropes on each side of the ship. His skin would become abraded and infected, and he often required hospitalization.

The most common punishment was by flogging with a nine-tailed whip (cat-o'-nine-tails) plaited with metallic beads or pieces of wire. In a fleet at anchor, the punishment was carried out in a longboat, the victim tied to a wooden upright, and the boat rowed from ship to ship. As it approached, the crew of a ship was drummed into formation to watch the spectacle of the flogging, the punishment being repeated at each ship. The surgeon was required to witness the punishment and had the power to discontinue it, if the victim's life was endangered. After punishment, the sailor was placed under the care of the surgeon, who washed the blood from the lash marks with brine and used salt packs as dressing, presumably to prevent infection. Months of hospitalization would be needed before recovery, the victim bearing the scars for the rest of his life.

Discipline in the United States

Flogging of seamen and soldiers was a controversial issue in America, where it was deemed demeaning and contrary to the democratic ideals of the new country. The sentence of flogging with the "cat" in the U.S. Navy was limited to the orders of American captains and first lieutenants and then only after a court-martial.[4]

However, Tilton, who was surgeon general of the army after the Revolutionary War, believed democracy stopped with military service: "Whatever may be the form of government, whether monarchical or republican, the government of the army (navy) must be despotic."[5]

Baron Charles Dupin in France remarked on the many defeats of the French navy at the hands of the British. "It is discipline which has been and will be the instrument of the great success of the British Navy, and it has been the want of discipline that has been the ruin of the French Navy."[6] Another French patriot protested that "the naval defeats of the French Republic and later the Empire, and the annihilation of the French Navy, were not owing to any deficiency in the personal courage or national attitude, but to loose disciplines, want of practical experience and bad gunnery." *Liberté, egalité, et fraternité* were not conducive to naval victory.

Only the fear of the lash, some said, kept some sailors performing their duties. English sailors who signed on American vessels were said to become bullying and disruptive when no longer threatened with punishment.

Many sailors regarded the lesser punishments of polishing brass or special work details as more degrading than a flogging. An elderly sailor on an American ship was brought before the captain after committing an offense. The captain remarked that if it weren't for his gray hairs he would be flogged, but instead would be punished by extra details and shining equipment. The sailor stripped off his shirt and begged to have the nine tails rather than be mocked by the crew while polishing brass!

Two-thirds of American sailors, after serving for years, had never been touched with the lash. Some captains adopted a more democratic way of administering punishment, and asked crew members to decide it by vote. In one such case, a paper was delivered to the captain by the crew, recommending a dozen lashes "well laid on" followed by drinking a quart of sea water—a more drastic punishment than the captain was prepared to order. More crewmembers signed up with a captain known for his righteousness, although he used flogging, than with one who was easygoing and avoided it.

The Surgeon's View

If the sailor on shore leave were so unfortunate as to be captured by a navy impressment gang and lose his freedom, he tended to serve in a surly manner and sought every opportunity to desert and escape. If escape was impossible, he feigned illness. Caustics on the skin produced ulcers, drinking tobacco brought on severe abdominal cramps, pain, retching and vomiting, and a quickened pulse. The navy surgeon was well familiar with these deceptions, and after treatment and a reprimand, the victim was assigned the most disagreeable detail.

John Milne was a reformer as well as ship surgeon, and, aboard his East Indiaman, he mothered his crew as children. He wrote a series of letters to William Hunter, the medical consultant of the Board of Trade, suggesting measures to improve the life and health of seamen. He hoped his letters to Hunter would be brought to the attention of the board. In his letters he proposed that crews be better paid and that each crew member pay one shilling a month to the surgeon as health insurance. The East India Company paid ship surgeons five pounds a month and the extra money received from the crew would make the post more attractive.

Milne also suggested that the purser provide clothing for the crew to replace the tattered rags with which they came to sea and that the ship's officers inspect the crew for cleanliness. On sailing, he proposed that each crew member receive a personal supply of tea, sugar, and tobacco to improve his life at sea. Captains should be ordered to anchor vessels at sites that were cool and salubrious, to improve the health of the crew. The monotony of salted meats in the diet, he said, should be broken by frequent stops when passing cultivated islands to provide fresh foods.

Milne was also a moralist. He asked that captains deny crew members shore leave in ports where they repeatedly returned on board drunk or with venereal diseases.

Although William Hunter was also regarded as a reformer, it is not known whether he ever championed Milne's ideas. We do know that they were never put into effect at this time, but over the next hundred years these reforms and others were mandated in some countries. In the United

States, President Adams addressed the problem of the health of sailors by signing into law an act for the "Relief of Sick and Disabled Seamen" in 1798. Twenty cents per month was deducted from the salary of seamen to build hospitals and provide for medical care.

Surgeons Against Impressment

Impressment was a major contributing cause to the appalling incidence of disease in the navy, as well as being responsible for severe disciplinary measures, desertions, and incompetence, and this evil led to mutinous behavior. Surgeons had to struggle against ignorance, stupidity, and entrenched traditions of both sailors and commanders; the commanders believed that reducing the severity of punishment was a frivolous novelty that breached the concept of hardship thought necessary for valiant seamen.[7]

In 1797, at a general meeting of naval medical officers at which he first recommended uniforms for sailors, Trotter made an argument against impressment that was submitted to the Admiralty. To avoid disease and the addition of incompetent men to the roster of a crew and to reduce desertions, he recommended a voluntary system. To make this work, the pay scale would have to be improved and modification made of the disciplinary regulations. Under such a system improved health and a better esprit de corps could be expected.[8]

Chapter 9

Shipwrecks and Survivors

F ROM THE SIXTEENTH CENTURY ships spread their sails to visit re-mote and uncharted seas on voyages of exploration, conquest, or trade. Many never returned, the victims of fierce storms and hurricanes, native uprisings on remote islands, mutinies, or naval engagements; survivors in small boats pitted puny resources against the wind and sea in the struggle for life.

Drifting day after day in a small boat or raft is the ultimate test of the will to live. Rough seas and high winds, water-soaked clothing, snow and cold or the blistering rays of the tropical sun, in addition to water and food shortages, torment the survivor. In a crowded boat, very likely, he has not only to tolerate association with classes and temperaments different from his own but to cooperate with them, without a moment of privacy, with no end in sight.

For the modern shipwreck survivor fortunate enough to have them, there are weapons against hunger, thirst, bitter cold, or exhausting heat—concentrated food, distillation equipment, survival clothing, radio communications—thanks to modern science. However, survival science has not overcome the psychological stresses of living with diverse personalities, or separation from one's community. Science alone does not teach survivors to live and work with each other, to seek a group, not a personal, escape.

Shipwrecked sailors thrust into the sea must struggle against immersion in the water, exposure to the elements, thirst, hunger, and erosion of the will to survive. In the days of sail, a seaman adrift in temperate waters, clinging to a mast or spar, could survive up to three days, after which exhaustion would prove fatal. Actual survival time would depend on physical fitness, water temperature, wave height, adequacy of clothing, and the presence of sharks and other predators.

Absent modern survival equipment, for those in a small boat, the dominant early events are wetness and cold. Shivering can maintain body temperature for a while, but as core body temperature falls, shivering is replaced with a reluctance to move, drowsiness, torpor, and death. In the age of sail, seamen who outlived the cold faced horrible effects of wetness itself. Huddling in a water-logged, overloaded boat in which feet and legs were constantly wet, combined with the inability to freely move, caused a condition known as immersion feet. The legs and feet would swell and go numb from tissue stasis and distention of the veins; the overlying skin would become so macerated that boots had to be cut off, revealing spreading ulcerations of the skin that promptly became infected. Individuals so afflicted were unable to stand, and gangrene could result. In tropical seas going over the side for a swim would increase circulation and ameliorate immersion foot.[1] Water below 50 degrees Fahrenheit led to frostbite, causing tissue necrosis due to arterial inadequacy; at such temperatures swimming obviously had no benefit.

The Will to Survive

The psychology of survivors from a foundered vessel has been well described.[2] As a sinking ship lowered its boats, the crew has been described as being in a depersonalized state, performing their tasks automatically, as if each individual were not experiencing the event. A state of shock and amnesia for the experience was common. Seamen in a lifeboat have been described as doing their jobs and following commands in a normal way, but remembering nothing afterwards.

Immediate ambient dangers that beset sailors afloat on a raft or clinging to a spar included sharks, barracudas attacking limbs left hanging in the water, and Portuguese men-of-war (medusae) stinging the already sun-blistered skin. Time stood still, as they later described it. Events of their past lives played out in their minds in a period seemingly years long but really lasting only a few seconds—selected scenes passing in review. Not only did actual events play out, according to their reports, but imagined and denied fantasies were screened in their thoughts. Death was expected, and the thought of dying became pleasurable.[3]

At the end of several days in a small boat, as the chances of an early rescue dimmed, survivors were overcome with depression; conversation lagged as a dry mouth made speaking an effort. Thirst overshadowed all other thoughts.

If plucked from the sea and hauled aboard a raft or a small boat, the immediate response was elation, then sadness for lost companions.

The Importance of a Leader

At some point in the shipwreck ordeal, a leader of the group might emerge. He was not necessarily of the highest rank, but he had qualities that enabled him gradually to assume responsibility and be tacitly accepted by the rest. He gave orders that were obeyed without question, and his leadership was accepted because his confidence and ability gave hope of salvation to those around him.

In the absence of such a unifying individual, there was little hope of survival. Dissension, quarreling, asocial behavior, a psychology of "every man for himself and the group be damned" pervaded the boat, reducing everyone's prospects. Without a leader, low morale quickly spread, and arguments over the size of the rations meted out often erupted. Delirium was common, as was aggressive behavior, and could require restraint. On one occasion, a sixteen-year-old boy was forced to defend himself against his crazed partner for three days and nights, with an axe.

A character study of those individuals who became leaders showed them to have practiced high standards of conduct throughout their lives and as having adhered to a rigid social code; their lives had been lived "without emotional extravagance."[4] When such a leader was recognized, a feeling of comradeship and sacrifice bonded the group, and heroism and self-sacrifice became manifest.

Heroism among persons in such a predicament is not unusual, as witnessed by one story of a delirious sailor who kept slipping off a raft while his two companions repeatedly dived into shark-infested waters to rescue him. Even without such a motive, going over the side of a small boat into the sea is not necessarily a suicide of despair. It may be an act of altruistic heroism, a wounded or disabled person's deliberate sacrifice to conserve a water ration for those more likely to outlast the wait for rescue.

Thirst

Eleven days approaches the record time for a lifeboat occupant to survive without drinking water.[5] The blood of sea birds, hand caught, has been drunk, as well as the blood of dead companions. In desperation, some have drunk urine, but this could have provided little relief because of its chemical nature and the scanty amount excreted by a dehydrated person.

Knowing that drinking seawater meant certain death, some drank it intentionally as a subtle form of suicide.

Distillation devices had been invented—the heat from the sun focused on a copper vessel of seawater—but were not available in small boats.[6] Sir Richard Hawkins, as early as the seventeenth century, wrote of a distillation device on board his ship.

> Although our fresh water had fayled us many days before we saw the shore by reason of our long navigation and the excessive drinking of the sicke and diseased, yet with an invention I had on my shippe, I easily drew out of the water of the sea, sufficient quantity of fresh water to sustain my people with little expense . . . for with foure bettels of wood I stilled a hogshead of water and therewith dressed the meat for the sicke and whole. The water so distilled we found wholesome and nourishing.[7]

By 1768 new distillation devices could produce forty-two gallons of fresh water in five hours—not much, but life-saving. A kettle was boiled and a musket barrel used as a condenser to funnel the water to a second kettle. The heat also killed any bacteria in the water.[8]

Hunger

If drinking water was available, hunger increased for thirty-six to seventy-two hours but gradually waned. Death from hunger would occur before signs of scurvy, which would develop in two to four weeks without fresh food. Attempts to catch fish with a hook and line were frustrating. A small fish hooked would be swallowed by a larger fish and the line would snap. A fish spear or a small-caliber shotgun provided more fish and also birds.[9] Even in a large vessel, death from hunger was not often recorded.

The crew of Lord Anson's fleet demonstrated the difficulties of survival. HMS *Wager*, one of the eight ships in Lord Anson's fleet circumnavigating the world in 1749, was severely damaged in a series of storms crossing Cape Horn through the Straits of Le Maire. The crew of the *Wager* had plenty of water from rain, ice, and snow, but food ran out as she floated aimlessly until repaired, with crewmembers dying from hunger. One of the crew with a grim sense of humor recorded the death of the purser, the noncommissioned officer who normally controlled the food supply, from starvation. "Wednesday, the 6th departed this life Mr. Thomas Harvey, the purser; he died a skeleton for want of food; this gentleman, probably the first purser belonging to His Majesty's Navy that ever perished with hunger."[10]

The sea in the *Wager's* crossing of Cape Horn was so violent that the incessant rolling of the ships made it impossible to stand on deck. Crew members were washed overboard, others dashed against masts and cabins. Fractured bones and a dislocation of the neck had to be treated. The snow and cold froze the rigging, making the sails brittle sheets of ice. Wet clothing froze on the men attempting to go aloft. When the cold weather subsided, dense fog rolled in and the fleet was separated, firing their guns in a desperate effort to locate each other. Two of the ships turned back. Scurvy then made its appearance, and thirty-four men died of this disease on a single ship, as they tried to reach their rendezvous at Juan Fernandez Island, off the west coast of Chile.

Another ship of Anson's fleet, the *Gloucester,* was dismasted, drifting and thought lost. Three-fourths of her crew were buried at sea, most because of scurvy, and not a man aboard was fit for duty. The rest of the fleet had reached Juan Fernandez Island and had access to fresh food. They combed the sea for the lost *Gloucester* and finally located it. The fresh food supplies from the relief vessel saved the lives of most of the *Gloucester's* remaining crew, but even with fresh greens, mortality continued for twenty days, six to eight dying daily.

Castaways

On Juan Fernandez island, the *Gloucester's* crew had found wild goats with slit ears and other signs of habitation that were thought to be the work of Alexander Selkirk, Defoe's inspiration for *Robinson Crusoe,* who had lived on it thirty-two years before.[11]

Selkirk had been put ashore after a dispute with his captain; his only possessions were a sea chest, the clothes he was wearing, a flintlock, a pound of gunpowder, a flint and steel, tobacco, a hatchet, knife, kettle, Bible, and other books, plus navigation instruments. After four years of survival due to his ingenuity, he was returned to England by a passing ship and was interviewed by Richard Steele for a magazine article on which Defoe based his book.[12]

Richard Clarke

In 1583, Richard Clarke, master of the ship *Admiral,* was shipwrecked with sixteen men crowded into a small boat near St. John's, Newfoundland. The one oar aboard was used as a rudder and a sail rigged. Another officer aboard suggested that they draw lots to choose four men to be thrown overboard to lighten the craft. Master Clarke, now the accepted leader, replied, "No, we will live together and die together."

When asked how far it was to shore, Clarke confidently assured the crew that they were within "two or three score of leagues," knowing well that they were much farther from shore than that. The weather was terrible; they saw the sun on one day only, and there were no stars to guide them at night. But Clarke was able to infuse the will to live. Several days out, after the death of several crewmembers, all desired to die, but Clarke again assured them they would sight land in a few days. If they didn't, he said, they could throw him overboard. Land was sighted the next day.[13]

Cannibalism

A different situation was reported in 1710, when Captain John Deane and his crew were shipwrecked on Boone Island off the coast of Maine. Two men had died, and no strong personality emerged. When the pangs of hunger became acute and after a night of wrangling and rationalizations, the majority voted to eat their dead companions. Some refused but relented the following day. They were described by their rescuers as having lost their natural dispositions and looked wild, fierce, and barbarous as a result of their cannibalism.[14]

Even more shocking behavior occurred on the American brigantine *Peggy* in 1765. The captain relinquished his command to the mob psychology of his crew. On the twenty-fourth of October, the *Peggy* was returning from Fayal in the Azores with a cargo of wine and spirits bound for New York, when she encountered severe storms in the North Atlantic that dismasted her and sprung several leaks. Totally disabled, she drifted out of control during the entire month of November, with the crew breaking into the hold and in a state of chronic intoxication. This seemed to appease their hunger for a time, but they then resorted to eating leather and candles. Captain Harrison withdrew and remained ill in his quarters, and the men assumed command. Then hunger was so acute that on January thirteenth, they told the captain they were going to draw lots, kill a man, and cannibalize him.

Harrison refused to consider this plan, but the men drew lots, which were probably rigged, and the unfortunate victim was the captain's black servant. By 26 January another drawing was made and another man selected, but they were rescued on 30 January before the crew could act.[15]

One Voyage, Two Mutinies

Another extreme example of an incompetent leader was that of Captain Cheap of the *Wager*, one of the ships in Anson's fleet, circumnavigating the world. During the ordeal traversing the Straits of Le Maire, Cheap had spent much of his time in his cabin withdrawing himself from the struggle and permitting his officers to assume command. On entering the Pacific after emerging from the straits, they sought a harbor to repair the damage inflicted by the storms and struck a reef near the shore, where the ship settled.

Cheap was unable to control the crew, who broke into the liquor closet and soon became drunk and disorderly—and also mutinous. Cheap fled to the shore in a small boat, soon followed by the crew. They claimed, now that the ship had sunk, that they were no longer bound to obey the captain. Cheap being unable to rise to the occasion, the crew accepted as their leader a midshipman named Cozens, who decided to sail the long-boat back to Brazil, although Cheap wanted to sail to Juan Fernandez Island and rendezvous with Anson.

Abandoning Cheap, who was no more than a prisoner, and his allies, the crew sailed for Brazil in the longboat—not, however, before Cheap had shot and mortally wounded Cozens. Cheap refused to allow the surgeon to aid the wounded Cozens, who suffered a lingering death before the eyes of the crew.

Two months later, Cheap and eleven remaining loyal supporters sailed north in the repaired yawl but were forced back due to bad weather. With the help of some local Indians, Cheap and his supporters then set sail for Chiloe Island off the coast of Chile. Putting into an island for the night, Cheap awoke the next morning and found that seven of the previously loyal crew had taken the boat and left him stranded with four companions. One of those stranded was the surgeon, Elliott, who died several days later. Cheap with his remaining three companions finally reached Chiloe Island with the help of the Indians and later returned to Britain. It is not often that a captain endures two mutinies in a single voyage.[16]

Captain Bligh

Survivorship is well recorded on one of the longest trips in an open boat by Captain William Bligh of the HMS *Bounty*, sailing in a launch twenty-three feet long with a beam of six feet, nine inches, which was crowded and low in the water with eighteen seamen, sailing from Tafoa, near Tahiti to the Island of Timor in Indonesia, a distance of 3,618 miles over a period of forty-one days.

The mutineers who seized the *Bounty* had allowed them no firearms and limited provisions. As the longboat pulled away from the *Bounty*, it carried twenty-eight gallons of water, 150 pounds of bread, a tool chest, twine, cordage, sails, and a quadrant. At the last minute, the mutineers threw four cutlasses into the launch. The course was WNW looking for Fiji. They did not have a timepiece or any charts. To estimate their speed, they constructed a log line, which is a rope knotted at regularly spaced intervals which, cast astern, allowed them to estimate the number of seconds it took to pay it out, timed by a pulse rate.

The carpenter used the seats to elevate the freeboard, and canvas was stretched over part of the boat to collect rain water and to protect them from the sun. Waves breaking over the side of the heavily over-crowded boat necessitated continuous bailing.

They landed at various islands, including Tofoa in the Friendly Islands, for fresh greens, coconuts, and water and also at an unidentified island they named Restoration Island. However, having lost a crewmember killed by the natives at Tofoa, they were cautious about landing on the many islands they passed in their defenseless condition.

Bligh, with his dominating personality, was the unquestioned leader and was rarely challenged. One man "with a mutinous look" went to him, saying he was as good as the captain and would no longer take orders. Bligh gave him a cutlass and dared him to duel with him, at which time the crewman withdrew. On another occasion, a crewman sent to collect birds' eggs concealed some on his person. Bligh personally gave him a thrashing.[17]

Hunger, not thirst, was their main problem. They had poor luck fishing but did catch some sea birds by hand. Bligh encouraged his men to dip their clothes in salt water and then to put them on. He firmly believed that the salt in the water would be removed by the skin as a dialyzing membrane and the fresh water absorbed into the body.

All aboard were weak and emaciated from lack of food, and keeping under way was a painful problem. They all complained of stiffness in attempting to move, dizziness, and constipation, but no one developed scurvy and no fever or disease occurred among them. They were isolated from outside sources of infection until they landed at Timor, at which time disease and fever spread and one man died.[18]

Bligh held his lifeboat crew together by personal force, fear, and the absence of anyone strong enough to challenge his decisions after the mutiny. Bligh was an efficient captain and a skillful navigator, who had the personality and talent to hold a crew together under trying circumstances.

Much has been written about Bligh. To some he was a tyrant and sadist, to others a brilliant officer challenged by a crew that couldn't face the realities of life in eighteenth-century England after spending six months of idyllic repose in a tropical island paradise with compliant women and girls as companions.

Bligh entered the navy through "the hawse pipe" at the lowest level and was from obscure parentage. He matured under the guidance of Captain Cook on the *Resolution* as sailing master at the early age of twenty-three.

To understand Bligh, one must acknowledge the role that Cook played in forming his leadership style. Cook was a father figure to his crew, attending to their comforts, diet, and health. He was especially proud of his sailing around the world over three years in which he lost only four men—only one from sickness. He derived more satisfaction from the health record of his crew than from his many discoveries and his contributions to navigation and cartography. When Cook was killed in Hawaii on his third voyage, his crew wept unashamedly, stating they had lost their father, and the sailor who deserted him when he was attacked was treated as a pariah with whom the crew would not associate. Cook never made any mention of aberrant behavior by Bligh, and in fact recommended that Bligh be promoted to a lieutenant.

Bligh's appointment as captain of the HMS *Bounty* was due to Sir Joseph Banks, the prominent naturalist who accompanied Cook on his first voyage of exploration. Banks had no discrediting remarks to make about Bligh, either.

The Admiralty did have some records alleging that Bligh treated his crew harshly, yet they reappointed him as captain on several assignments after the mutiny, and he served with Nelson at the Battle of Copenhagen and received Nelson's thanks for his support. Later, he served two years as governor of New South Wales in Australia, where his personality led to several confrontations with the merchants and the military that resulted in the termination of his post. He achieved the rank of rear admiral before he died.

The Twentieth Century

Misadventure on the open sea is timeless; it is the same now in its terror and isolation as it was thousands of years ago. It is also easy to forget that ships worked under sail, in commerce, in battle, and in exploration, well into the twentieth century. Captain Foster of the *Trevassa* and Sir Ernest Shackleton of the *Endurance* met disaster on the same terms—except mutiny—that confronted Captain Bligh.

The Trevassa

The crew of the *Trevassa* traveled 1,700 miles in the Indian Ocean in 1911 before being rescued. She sank in a storm, and the crew escaped in two lifeboats, one commanded by Captain Foster, the other in charge of the chief officer. Each boat was twenty-six feet long, with a beam of eight feet. The two boats hovered near the sinking *Trevassa* until she finally submerged, as a murmur arose from the boats, "She's gone."

The officers put everyone to work and so were able to lift their spirits. The boats had to be headed up to the mountainous waves, sea anchors had to be contrived, provisions carefully stowed and secured, and lines laid out to link the two lifeboats. Several days out, they agreed to part company, as they had spent too much time each morning looking for each other after separation during the night.

Captain Foster had all the provisions in his boat brought aft under his personal safeguard. Anything that could be used as a weapon, such as oarlocks and knives, was passed aft to be under his control.

Rations were carefully doled out under the scrutiny of all hands, to satisfy their need for parity, and no one was favored. Twenty days later, rations were reduced. One man gave up and harangued the crew, sure they would never be rescued, while the rest of the crew listened dejectedly. Captain Foster, in reply, used his leadership position to cheer them, confidently saying that they were on course for Rodriguez Island in the Mauritius group of islands near Madagascar and that their chances of being rescued were excellent.

Illusions occurred almost nightly; the men would see what they thought were lights or flares that were in fact only beams from a distant brilliant star. Each boat, now sailing separately, did have a sextant and charts. However, navigation proved to be a problem, as neither had a chronometer. They resolved it by sailing north until they reached the latitude of Rodriguez Island and then sailing westward along this latitude until the island would appear.

Stiffness and soreness from lack of movement tormented them. To alleviate thirst, they were encouraged to soak rags in the sea water and place them on their nostrils but were severely cautioned not to swallow any sea water. One man drank some sea water anyway and then begged for an extra water ration because of the great thirst that followed, but he was denied it. This posed an interesting problem. Should ill survivors be given extra water rations?

Water was issued two hours after the noon sighting of the sun. Foster made his calculations deliberately, with all eyes fixed upon him; he learned to smile confidently and nod agreeably in answer to their questioning looks. The two hours following the sighting was an eternity, and the men begged for a few drops of their ration before time, which was always denied.

Early on they managed a cheerful attitude, as if they were on a yachting cruise, but as the days passed gloom settled over the crew. Captain Foster kept up the chatter and assured them that they were entering the trade routes to the Mauritius and that they would be picked up at almost any time. All looked haggard and emaciated after two weeks, but aside from some boils, the health of all remained good.

With little to do except occasionally to change a sail, the survivors lapsed into a semicomatose condition with dreams of home, only to be brought back to reality by the noise of a flapping sail or a wave-top breaking over the side.

When the wind dropped, Foster had them use the oars, not because they made any headway but to give the men a job to do. It improved morale to be working as a team.

On the seventeenth day the first man died and, a day later, the second. All the survivors were drawn and weakened. At the start it took one man to hoist the sail; later it required three.

Rain squalls gave everyone an extra drink. Canvas covers were of little use to catch water, as it never rained enough to wash out the encrusted salt in the cover. Rainwater was best collected by letting the water run down the head and pointing the beard into a cup to collect a luxurious drink.

About this time, several crewmembers caused trouble and refused to do their share of the work, but most remained loyal, singing together with cracked voices to keep up their spirits.

Twenty-two days after the *Trevassa* sank, Foster's boat reached Rodriguez Island, having covered 1,556 miles.

The second boat, under the command of the chief officer, missed Rodriguez but made Mauritius. Control was not as strict on this boat; they soaked their biscuits in sea water and seven men died. One was lost overboard, and one died just after landing. This boat had covered 1,747 miles in twenty-four days.[19]

Shackleton's Voyage on the Lifeboat James Caird

The *Endurance,* which bore Sir Ernest Shackleton and his crew to Antarctica, was a sailing ship with auxiliary steam. The lifeboat, *James Caird,* in which he and five of his crew made their most heroic voyage, was propelled by sail.

When the *Endurance* became locked in the ice off Antarctica, the dreams and hopes of a successful mission were dashed. There was to be no glory, no discoveries, only the test of survival. Shackleton would appear to have faced a serious morale problem. But, like James Cook, Shackleton prided himself in the safe return of his crew. He consulted with his men and sought their opinions each time they faced a dangerous situation and a decision had to be made. (In any event, mutinous behavior seldom develops in an all-volunteer crew camped on a moving ice floe with no hope of outside help.)

Shackleton can be faulted for poor planning, and the expedition itself had no scientific goals. It was an adventurous stunt to cross the Antarctic continent and to rendezvous with another ship on the opposite side—a challenge for the sake of challenge. But his eight-hundred-mile trip to South Georgia Island on a twenty-two-and-a-half-foot lifeboat was not a stunt but true heroism as he sought help to rescue his stranded crew. With five crewmembers and basic navigation instruments dependent on fixing the sun and stars—which were obscured for thirteen of the seventeen days of the voyage through treacherous seas in stormy weather—his voyage is a feat equal to or surpassing that of Bligh.

Even after reaching South Georgia Island, his task remained incomplete, as he was unable to convince the British Admiralty, beset with a world war, to send a rescue ship. To save his crew stranded on Elephant

Island, he continued his efforts with mounting frustration to arrange for a rescue vessel, until the Chilean government made a concession.[20]

Offshore Wrecks

Between 1789 and 1800, 2,957 British ships were lost at sea, according to Lloyd's List, and of these, 652 were dashed against the rocky British shoreline, with great loss of life. In coastal villages the fishermen preferred to drink their ale in the warm local pub rather than risk their lives at sea as a storm drove a vessel against the rocks. There were exceptions, and in the Yorkshire village of Redcar the customs house officer proudly displayed the names of two hundred seamen saved between 1800 and 1824. The drama of lifeboats was well described in the record.

As the lifeboat was launched, the breakers flooded the boat, to the agony of the rescuers' families, watching on shore. The heavy seas broke oars as the rescuers approached a vessel, the hull disappearing with each heavy wave and the terrified crew clinging to the rigging. When, after they had achieved the rescue and returned to shore, another person appeared on the rigging, the original lifeboat crew, numbed with the cold, was eagerly replaced with fresh volunteers.[21]

The Humane Society in Britain, in an effort to reduce the loss of seamen from offshore wrecks, offered a prize for the best solutions to these problems in 1799. This competitive prize was won by Dr. Anthony Fothergill, who published a small book on rescuing survivors with many answers.

Fothergill illustrated his recommendations by describing the wreck of the *Juno,* which left a Captain McKay and thirteen survivors afloat in a small boat with limited water over a period of twenty-three days. This captain showed little understanding of survival techniques. They drank seawater and chewed on lead from the wreck, believing it to cause salivation. Men who could not swim fell overboard. No leader emerged, and no hope of rescue prevailed among the survivors. Fortunately, rescue did occur, so their experience could benefit others.

Fothergill suggested that, for a start, better understanding of weather forecasting should be sought. He described how the natives in different parts of the world understood local weather patterns and said that mariners would be wise to consult them. Spanish seamen sailing in the West Indies quickly learned the Indian term "hurricane" and took appropriate action. The Caribs of St. Dominica and St. Vincent, he stated, could anticipate, with accuracy, the approach of a hurricane when they saw a blood-like redness to the setting sun and a halo around a full moon, with blurred stars and a gloomy sky in the northwest. When the barometric pressure fell, wells and caverns sent forth a hollow sound; the sea calmed and a rank odor arose from the water. When the wind veered from the northwest to east or southeast, the storm would end.

Fothergill also urged that all seamen be taught to swim and that whenever possible crews should go over the side of the small boat to remain in the water for a brief period. Like Bligh and many others, he thought that clothing soaked in seawater allowed the lymphatic system and the skin to act as a filtering membrane to remove the salt and let desalinated water enter the body. Benjamin Franklin also subscribed to this theory.

Rescue Boats

Fothergill also suggested that ships be inspected for safety and that lightning rods be mounted on masts (another Franklin recommendation). Most important, however, were his comments about the people on shore viewing the death struggles of a ship being dashed against the reef in a heavy sea.

The crowds that assembled to view the spectacle were drawn to the cliffs for two reasons. Some came to plunder the wreck when it was finally cast ashore, and in some cases even to lure vessels to the rocks with lanterns on shore to misguide the mariners. A second group wrung their hands in anguish and hoped that there was something that they could do to help. It was for this latter group that Fothergill suggested boats so constructed that they could be launched in heavy weather and crews trained to man these boats, with appropriate rewards to inspire the local fishermen. Fothergill did not accept his monetary award for his essay but returned it to the Humane Society.

The aim was to construct an unsinkable lifeboat. In 1784, Lionel Lufkin started with a yawl and added a projecting gunwale of cork, nine inches wide amidships. He also constructed a watertight compartment at each end. The boat was tested and behaved well, but no one evinced any interest, not even the Admiralty.

The first lifeboat to rescue a survivor was a boat planned and constructed by a landlubber named Greathead and launched in 1790. It was made buoyant by a fender of cork twelve inches wide from stem to stern and used seven hundred pounds of cork. Thirty feet long, with a beam of ten feet and a high prow and stern, it had three sliding keels to allow it to be pushed from the beach to the surf, and it was pulled by ten oars. It lay in readiness on shore, suspended by slings from twelve-foot wheels. This craft first saw action in 1791 and continued its good work, saving many crews. By 1803 Greathead had built thirty-one such rescue boats. Self-righting and self-bailing boats were still to be developed.[22]

Firing a mortar ball several hundred yards distant was also first described at this time. The ball with a light rope attached to it was fired across the deck of a distressed ship and used to haul a heavier rope on board. The rope could be used as a bridge by individuals lashed to it or as a guide for a small boat.[23]

Much later, lifeboat stations dotted the British coast, manned by a volunteer organization that is still operative today.

Chapter 10

Marine Medicine in the United States

THE AMERICAN REVOLUTION began without an established navy. However, each coastal colony had excellent sailors and shipwrights, as well as ship suppliers. The rebels well understood that, if the struggle for American independence were to be successful, naval and maritime support, domestic and foreign, was urgent. Certainly, without the assistance of the French navy at the mouth of the Chesapeake Bay in 1778, the brilliant encirclement and defeat of Cornwallis at Yorktown could never have been accomplished.

Each of the American colonies had maintained seaports for almost one hundred years for coastal, Caribbean, and transatlantic trade. Ships hastily built in America now had to transport military supplies for the use of the Continental Army and the provincial militias. Privateers were also fitted out to harry British merchantmen and troop transports, which sought the protection of warships that Britain could ill afford to spare from her European wars.

The increase in maritime activity in America required many more doctors to act as surgeons or surgical mates, but they were in short supply. There were only two medical schools, the College of Philadelphia and Kings College in New York, each graduating twenty to thirty doctors a year. Most practicing doctors never went to medical school and were trained in an apprenticeship to an established physician for two to five years. Both the graduates and the apprentices preferred to practice near their families in their home communities, where they were much in demand. Moreover, the wages offered a maritime surgeon and a surgical mate were not enticing (fifty dollars a month, plus rations for a surgeon; thirty-nine dollars a month for a surgical mate). The average shore doctor charged one dollar for a house visit and could earn about two hundred dollars a month. On the other hand, prize money for a captured vessel could provide a small fortune. A good meal in this period cost eighty cents.

The Continental Congress, recognizing the importance of maritime support for its armies, passed the first naval appropriation bill in November 1775, marking $100,000 to be used for armament on thirteen vessels. In the same act, rules about the sharing of prizes and treatment of prisoners were also laid down. Captains and crews were entitled to one-third of the cargo of a captured vessel. Of this one-third, the captain received six shares, each man one share, and the surgeon four shares. The surgeon's wages were set at twenty-one and one-third dollars per month. For comparison, the captain received thirty-two dollars and seamen and marines received six and two-thirds dollars per month.

Congress spelled out the rules to be observed by captains of American warships and privateers. "If you or any of your officers or crew shall in cold blood kill, maim, or by torture or otherwise cruelly, inhumanely, and contrary to usage and the practice of civilized Nations in War, treat any Person or Persons surprised in the Ship or Vessel you shall take, the Offender shall be severely punished." These regulations were copied from orders to British captains issued by the Admiralty.[1]

The View from England

During the American Revolutionary War there were 89,000 British regulars and 2400 Hessians fighting alongside the Tories against "the rebels." Later, this expeditionary force was reduced to 56,000 as the tensions in Europe mounted and troops were withdrawn.

Great Britain's logistical problems of transporting manpower, artillery, munitions, and horses in convoy three thousand miles across the ocean, in a voyage of three to six weeks, with French and rebel ships ready to prey upon stragglers en route, seemed insurmountable. Then, once the troops and supplies reached the American shore, they had to be distributed over a thousand-mile coastline between Maine and Georgia.

Supplies were necessary for the boat crews, as well as the transported marines and regulars. They all crowded together on armed merchantmen of two to three hundred tons, usually traveling in convoys, shepherded by men-of-war, but at other times alone. The holds were converted to living quarters and subdivided into tiers, each tier holding six men packed together spoonwise. At a command from the end man of "about face," everyone turned to the opposite side.

With so many people on board, the usual food problems escalated. Biscuits were crawling with maggots, pork was streaked with decay, and on opening a water cask, foul smells from contaminants were vented; dysentery spread throughout the ship. There were no fresh greens or lime juice, and scurvy added to the misery. Smallpox and typhus fever rapidly spread because of the crowding and inability to isolate the sick. On one convoy bound for New York in 1779 with 3,868 personnel aboard, a hundred died during the crossing and 795 reported sick with typhus alone. On the ships' reaching New York, these diseases were quickly spread to troops on station, and six thousand were sent to improvised hospitals—commandeered houses, churches, and halls—to be treated for typhus by bleeding, purgatives, and various ineffective medicines.

Ships that dared to sail out of convoy in crossing the Atlantic were often attacked by American privateers and French men-of-war. In 1776 and again in 1780, American and French vessels successfully halted and captured British transports.

A guards officer described life aboard one of these transports: "Continued destruction in the foretops from the Atlantic storms, the pox above, the plague between decks, hell in the forecastle, the devil at the helm." As the passengers and crew crowded together for weeks, the men's tempers flared and their anger led to fights, duels, and suicides.[2]

There was only one fleet engagement in the Revolutionary War, on Lake Champlain, and Benedict Arnold, who happened to be an army general, built the Continental fleet that fought and lost it. While assembling his carpenters, rope makers, gunnery instructors, and other necessary personnel, Arnold asked the army's Dr. Jonathan Potts to send him some doctors. An American surgeon, Isaac Senter, had successfully treated Arnold's leg wound after the assault on Quebec, but Arnold either had a poor opinion of surgeons or couldn't resist a quip. In his letter to Potts he requested "any surgeon . . . who will answer to kill a man *secundum artem* [in the scientific method]."[3] After much delay, Dr. Francis Hagan, with Dr. McCrea as assistant, reported to Arnold.

The treatment of war casualties during the Revolutionary War, both in the army and navy, followed the recommendations made by John Jones, M.D., professor of surgery at King's College in New York City, who in 1775 published the first textbook of surgery and fractures in America as a manual to instruct the young military and naval surgeons in North America.[4]

After the Revolution

Directly following the cessation of hostilities between the United States and Britain, there was a rapid increase in the number of Yankee merchantmen, so that the American ensign was quickly introduced and recognized in harbors throughout the world. In Far Eastern and Chinese ports, the number of American ships equaled the British. In Whampoa, near Canton, China, in 1807, the American surgeon, Baldwin, counted twenty ships flying the American ensign anchored in this harbor.[5]

In 1798 President John Adams recognized the health problems of the thousands of American merchant seamen throughout the world and signed into law "An Act for the Relief of Sick and Disabled Seamen," providing them with marine hospitals, which later developed into the Public Health Service. Twenty cents was deducted each month from the salary of each seaman to build or rent hospitals and to pay for medical care. Castle Island in Boston Harbor was the first marine hospital, and Dr. Thomas Welch, a veteran of Lexington and Concord, was appointed as physician in charge in 1799. In 1807, Dr. Benjamin Waterhouse, who introduced the smallpox vaccine of Jenner into America, was made physician in charge of this marine hospital. Other hospitals were built, and the tax on seamen continued until 1884, at which time Congress made appropriations for the support of such hospitals.

The "Pseudo-War"

It was not long before the newly constituted United States Navy was challenged. The Atlantic and Mediterranean trade was charged with tension soon after the war, as the postwar treaty of friendship between the United States and France collapsed and French vessels sought to interdict American trade with Britain. When the new egalitarian government took control, the American treaty with France was scrapped. The Napoleonic dictatorship that followed did not recognize it, either. During the early years of Napoleon's rule, France proved to be most troublesome to American shipping, and an undeclared war or "pseudo-war" existed.

The first American warship, the *United States,* with fifty guns, was completed in 1797. Six additional warships were built in 1797 and 1798 to protect foreign trade, after Congress abrogated the Franco-American treaty in 1796 and ordered American captains to attack French vessels. The "pseudo-war" soon ended on 30 September 1800, when a new treaty was signed with France.

Edward Cutbush

Dr. Edward Cutbush graduated medical school in Philadelphia in 1794 and joined the navy after gaining much medical experience treating yellow fever in Philadelphia during the epidemic in 1793. In his naval journal he described treating dysentery, venereal disease, and fevers on board, but, like most medical graduates, he had a keen interest in natural philosophy extending beyond the practice of medicine.

One of Cutbush's enthusiasms was his theory about using water temperature to determine a ship's longitude, no reliable device for doing so being in existence at the time. He kept a "thermometrical journal" to record water temperature on his eastward and westward journeys. His theory depended on a set course for the Gulf Stream and other currents (which is not the case) and did not receive wide acceptance.[6] More valuable to us are his comments on preparing a ship for its inevitable wounded.

He vividly described the activity that took place on his frigate when a strange sail appeared on the horizon. When the drums beat to quarters, Cutbush and his surgical mates with their "loblolly boy"—the corpsman, so called for the "loblolly" gruel served to the sick—took their places in the cockpit (serving as the operating room and the dressing station); it was dark and stuffy, just above the hold and below the water line on the orlop—lowest—deck. This was the living quarters of the surgeon's mates, senior midshipmen, clerks, purser, and chaplain. The surgeon was quartered in the wardroom.

In preparation for battle, the mess table was lashed to the deck and used as an operating table. The purser and chaplain assisted the surgeon and his mates. Casks of water were in readiness. Instruments were laid out and covered with a cloth to conceal them from the eyes of frightened casualties. These included sets for amputation of limbs, trepanning skulls, soft tissue dissecting instruments, tenacula, needles armed with thread, tourniquets, ligatures, bandages, lint compresses, linen, skin plasters, retractors, thread, tape, splints, and gags to place in the mouths of patients under the knife. A tub of sand to catch the blood was available to keep the cockpit deck from becoming slippery. Each person was again instructed in his duties, and additional men were requested from the first mate to help carry the wounded.[7]

The tactics of naval warfare initially depended on long-range cannon that projected a twelve- to twenty-pound ball over a mile. For dueling at closer range, the carronade projected shot, weighing about twenty pounds, for a short distance, similar to a mortar. The ships were expertly maneuvered to take advantage of the wind, to avoid the enemy's fire, and to bear down on the enemy. After preliminary skirmishing, the ships closed in broadside to each other and fired rapidly. Men on deck were showered with wooden splinters from the mast and spars and metal parts from the rigging when the ball struck the ship. Canisters and grapeshot were anti-personnel weapons intended to burst upon the deck, sending glass, metal, and stones hurtling in all directions. Muskets, cutlasses, and pikes caused other wounds at closer range.[8]

Cutbush advised the surgeon to treat all patients without regard to rank. The patient's questions about his injury were to be answered to inspire confidence and a quick recovery: "When we are obliged to arm our hands with steel, shall we likewise steel our hearts and our brows with terror? Certainly not."[9]

If metal or wood splinters were in the wound, they were removed whenever possible, but extensive, time-consuming probing was discouraged. "There is only one good probing instrument that avoids damage to blood vessels and nerves—the index finger." To calm the trembling, shivering, apprehensive patient, often as young as sixteen years, opiates were to be given with brandy, but there was no anesthesia.

The small entrance wound of a musket ball was to be enlarged. Wounds were cleaned with a water-soaked sponge, bleeding stopped by pressure or a ligature, and the tourniquet reapplied if those measures failed. The surgeon would not amputate on the spot unless the indications were very clear, favoring instead to postpone the decision as long as possible.

After treatment, patients were removed from the cockpit to the adjacent gun room or the berth deck for observation, and the slightly wounded were ordered back to duty. If there was fever after surgery, Cutbush recommended a low diet and repeated bleedings as necessary. He believed that animal food was the best sustenance after wounding. Leeches were attached to the wound edges to reduce the swelling.

Tetanus (lockjaw) was the most feared complication, according to Cutbush, and always resulted in death. The tetanic symptoms of stiffness, facial grimacing, rigidity of the spine, and distortion of the limbs were palliated with calomel, opium, and cold baths.

Larrey, Napoleon's chief surgeon, treated all wounds with a hot cautery and claimed he could prevent tetanus. However, the use of hot oil and cautery applied to a wound had been severely criticized by Ambroise Paré over a hundred years earlier, and Cutbush's treatments were those used by the British. They were based upon the ideas of military and naval surgeons such as Paré, Pringle, Blane, Trotter, and LeDran, and those described by John Jones in his military manual for American surgeons. The wound was dressed, foreign material removed if accessible, but not cauterized.

U.S. Navy regulations in 1802 outlined the duties of the surgeon:

1. To inspect and take care of medical necessities on board.
2. To visit the sick on board twice daily or more often.
3. To consult with the surgeon of the squadron on difficult cases.
4. To submit a report to the captain daily.
5. To always be prepared for an engagement.
6. To keep a daybook of his activities and the names and treatment of those sick and dead.
7. To requisition stores for which he is responsible for the expenditure. This included medicines, equipment and instruments.

Cutbush, in his book published in 1808, *Preserving the Health of Soldiers and Sailors,* made recommendations to the surgeon regarding specific instruments and medicines needed on board.

Peter St. Medard

The day-to-day medical and surgical problems presented to the surgeon of a naval ship in this era come vividly alive in the medical log of surgeon Peter St. Medard of the 36-gun frigate *New York* on a sixteen-month cruise during the quasi-war with France. Over 50 percent of his patients suffered from catarrh, pulmonic diseases, and other upper respiratory complaints; 16 percent had diarrhea and dysentery; bilious disease, fevers, rheumatism, and venereal diseases accounted for 20 percent.

In the U.S. Navy, venereal disease victims were still punished by a five-dollar fine. The British had long ago rescinded any penalty or monetary payment for treatment of venereal disease, as they recognized that it led to concealment of the disease. In America, the fine was levied until 1840.

Some scurvy developed on the *New York* during the homeward journey to Washington. Treatment of scurvy provided by St. Medard included quinine, wine, elixir of vitriol, cinnamon, ginger root, and vinegar lemonade, which must have had no residual potency as it failed to cure the scorbutic seamen.

Of the 488 sick visits that St. Medard listed in the daybook, 6 percent were for injuries, including falls from rigging resulting in fractures and dislocations. On one occasion a major explosion on board killed three and burned many others.[10]

St. Medard's medicine chest included quinine (now used instead of cinchona bark) for fevers; for syphilis, mercury, plus an "abstemious diet" and topical application of caustics. Cholera was treated with rhubarb, calomel, and opium. Rheumatism was thought to be improved with opium and calomel. Ship fever (typhus) called for wine, quinine, and sprinkling vinegar in the living area daily. For each of these maladies, treatment included bleeding.

Other diseases included smallpox, which by this time was preventable by vaccination. Measles was treated with quinine and bleeding. Tuberculosis was recognized from the emaciation of the sailor, coughing of blood, and difficulty in breathing, for which no specific treatment was recommended. All three, of course, are highly communicable.

Quarantine

In his book, Cutbush had reiterated the suggestion of Lind that all recruits be isolated to determine if they harbored disease before being allowed to join their ship. Although it was still universally believed that disease was a result of toxic air, it was also recognized that a sick person could pass on his sickness to a healthy shipmate; thus the sick should be isolated and the clothing and bedding of a sick sailor who died was to be thrown overboard—or alternatively scrubbed and smoked before reuse.

When disease appeared and the cause and treatment were unknown, separation of the diseased from the healthy to prevent its spread had been successfully practiced for hundreds of years. The Italian city-states on the Adriatic Sea kept passengers and crew members suspected of illness from entering the community for an arbitrary forty days, the quarantenaria. It was a shotgun approach, but it worked.

The first federal quarantine laws in the United States were passed in 1796, and immediately raised the issue of the federal government trampling on states' rights, until Chief Justice John Marshall ruled that all matters of health were in the jurisdiction of the states. Yet, in 1878, Congress took the leading role to enforce quarantine laws, and the enforcing agency was the Marine Hospital Service of the United States Public Health Service.[11]

Discipline and Working Conditions of Sailors

Cutbush followed the recommendations of the British naval surgeon, Trotter, in suggesting that men selected for the military and naval services should ideally be between eighteen and forty years of age. He discussed proper clothing and a change to dry clothing; he recommended that the hair be cut short for sanitary purposes. He also advised discipline to fit the crime. Although flogging was accepted, the severe disciplinary measures of the British Navy were unnecessary, as impressment of seamen was never authorized in America (see chapter 8).

Flogging was abolished in the United States Navy in 1840.

Provisions and Sanitation

Cutbush synthesized the most recent medical information and placed it in book form to make it available to surgeons in the newly established U.S. Navy.

Discussing water on shipboard, Cutbush said it should be strained through sand to prevent a stale taste, and marshy water boiled to kill the animaliculae. Vinegar was also added to drinking water for this purpose. This is an improvement over Trotter's suggestion to char the inside of the water cask, but what is most interesting about Cutbush's observations is that he thought creatures swimming or floating in the water were associated with disease. Cutbush didn't explicitly say this, and probably he continued to believe that disease arose from toxic air or water, but he seems to have sensed that drinking water containing swimming objects was unsanitary, if not the cause of disease.

His advice regarding newly commissioned ships was to dry them thoroughly between decks by lighting fires and then whitewash the interior planking. Even the gravel of the ballast was to be washed and cleaned in an effort to avoid the stench of the bilge.

Air was correctly understood to be composed of oxygen, nitrogen, and carbon dioxide, but, of course, those putrid elements from noxious effluvia could toxify it and cause disease. Land air, too, could be toxic, and smelled differently from sea air; one could recognize it up to three or four miles before making shallow soundings. A spaniel on board was said to have smelled land and barked continuously, running to the gangplank, four days before land was sighted.

In the harbor, Cutbush warned, ports should be closed when an offshore breeze is blowing air over marshy areas that contained "effluvia." Anchoring in a marshy harbor should be at least a mile and a half from the nearest shore (as it happens, about the range of a mosquito). The preferable anchorage should have a landward-directed breeze. Cutbush also recommended lime juice, as used in the British Navy to prevent scurvy, but exercises and cheerfulness were also said to prevent this disease.

At this juncture of history, cleanliness, fresh food, strict sanitation, and quarantine of disease were recognized as necessary to prevent sickness, although the specifics of transmission and the causes of disease remained unknown until much later.[12] The cleanliness and order of American frigates were said to surpass the vessels of all other nations, even Great Britain. Officers from other nations visiting the *Constellation* while in port in Italy were quick to remark upon her "spit and polish."[13]

Cutbush itemized the daily duties of the surgeon in his book. They included the surgeon's selecting and bringing with him to his ship his personal instruments and medications. Once a day, too, he sent his loblolly boy throughout the ship ringing a bell to advertise he was having sick call. After this he attended those in the sick berth and made two lists of those who were excused from duty; one was given to the captain, the other was sent to the binnacle for the officer of the day.[14]

War Against the Barbary Pirates

The quasi-war with France had just been settled when the young republic found itself in another naval war. Attacks on American and European shipping by the Barbary pirates from Morocco, Algiers, Tunisia, and Tripoli increased, and a truce between the United States and Tripoli signed in 1795 was no longer in effect. Much of the population of North Africa had been expelled from Spain three hundred years earlier and continued to hold a hatred for all Europeans.

American ships in the Mediterranean and even in the Atlantic approaches were being captured and the crews sold into slavery. The *Oswego,* a recently built ship, sailed from New York to Cork, Ireland, on 8 January 1800. Her next port of call was Madeira, but as a result of navigation errors, she was wrecked off the Barbary Coast in northwest Africa. In a detailed journal, Capt. Judah Paddock described how he and his crew were sold into slavery by the Arabs and then resold to another bidder, detailing their suffering until they were rescued by the British consul in Magadore.[15]

British and French vessels were also attacked by the Barbary pirates, but these nations were locked in a war, accepted the hazards, and did not retaliate. However, President Jefferson was determined to put an end to this plundering and ordered the American fleet to neutralize the threat. The fleet included the frigates *United States, Constellation,* and *Constitution,* which were the nucleus of the navy. Additional frigates were to be constructed so that sufficient sea power was available to blockade Tripoli.

The Barbary pirates in their small boats could not stand off the cannonade of a frigate. Instead they closed in and boarded the ship by dropping their long lateen sails across the deck of the enemy, scrambling aboard by using the sail as a boarding net. Edward Cutbush at that time was surgeon on the *Constellation* and was ordered to report as surgeon for the newly built *Philadelphia,* which was in readiness to sail for North Africa. He was unable to reach her before she sailed, and Dr. Jonathan Cowdery was sent in his place.

Dr. Cowdery's Letters

During her patrols along the North African coast, the *Philadelphia* went aground four miles from the town of Tripoli, and after a battle she was seized by the enemy and her crew captured. Dr. Cowdery, in two letters smuggled out of Tripoli, described the plight of the American captives. One letter, which described his capture, was sent to his father and is dated November 7, 1804. A second, shorter letter was mailed to a Dr. Mitchell on 24 November 1804. His diary also described his capture.[16]

In his description of his capture, he told of being led off the *Philadelphia* by a Tripolitan officer holding a rifle in one hand and ransacking his pockets of ten dollars with the other. Some gold sewn in his pockets was not discovered by his captors, but they did take his box of medications and surgical instruments and clubbed his head just before reaching shore. Cowdery and the American officers were initially imprisoned in a castle. He wrote of "the dreary cells of a castle, the gloomy halls of which bespeak the miseries of Christian slaves who erected them under the lash of tyrants, the glimmering light of which is admitted through an iron grating."

His instruments and medication were soon returned to him by the local ruler, the bashaw, who alternately befriended him when he provided treatment for the bashaw's family and harshly judged him when his mood changed.

Cowdery and the other officers were later incarcerated in a house near the harbor, from the roof of which they could witness the excitement of the population looting the *Philadelphia.* They witnessed Tripolitans wearing officers uniforms and carrying looted goods. Cowdery was able to single out a renegade Scotsman who was the Tripolitan admiral.

The bashaw was devoted to his children, so that when one child became seriously ill, Cowdery was sent for and asked to treat the child, who recovered. In appreciation, the bashaw provided him with a servant and a horse and permitted him to visit his gardens and orchard. On another occasion he treated one of the bashaw's two wives. In becoming indispensable to the bashaw, Cowdery realized he was jeopardizing his chances of freedom. He was told by his captor that he wouldn't take a ransom of twenty thousand dollars for his release.

Cowdery ministered to the 360 crewmen of the *Philadelphia,* who were treated as slaves rather than prisoners and were harnessed to carts, hauling rocks to repair the harbor fortification. They were beaten and kept on a starvation diet. Cowdery remonstrated with the bashaw, who claimed that he knew nothing of it and would act to improve the lot of the seamen, but there was no change.

On 16 February 1805, the officers were alerted by great excitement about the harbor and learned that two ships flying British colors were entering the harbor. About midnight they were awakened by shouting and screaming and saw crowds running through the streets. The *Philadelphia* was ablaze. Cowdery described how the officers were choked with emotion and national pride, lessening the rigors of their captivity.

During the night, Lieutenant Stephen Decatur, with a commando crew, had boarded the *Philadelphia,* and succeeded in setting her afire. Admiral Nelson called Decatur's action "the most bold and daring of the age."[17]

Many of the enemy aboard the *Philadelphia* were burned, and Cowdery described their treatment of burns, which consisted of anointing the burned area with honey and leaving the wound exposed. Periodically, fine powder of lead was sprinkled onto the wound until it healed. High concentrations of lead must have entered the circulation to slowly poison the wounded.

Meanwhile, American diplomatic efforts continued to free the hostages. In a strategic move, the Americans decided to support and provide an army for the bashaw's brother, who had claimed the title and had been exiled. (Another contesting brother had been killed by the bashaw.) The bashaw had demanded $1,690,000 in ransom for the hostages but, fearing an invasion by his brother's army, accepted $60,000. After sixteen months of captivity, the Americans were freed.

Cowdery had a long tenure as a naval surgeon. He joined the navy in 1799 and remained in the service until 1852.

Reforming Naval Medicine: William Barton

It is not often that a naval medical officer subjected to court-martial proceedings becomes chief of the Bureau of Medicine and Surgery. Young Doctor William Barton, appointed as surgeon in 1809, was a novice in the navy and disdainful of many of his superiors. Because of his severe criticism of the conditions at the navy yard at Philadelphia, he was brought up on charges of tarnishing the reputation of his superiors in 1818. He had printed articles describing navy personnel huddled in miserable houses without provisions on the navy bases. The court heard the charges and his arguments and sidestepped the issue by admitting that conditions were bad and that no refutation of the charges was necessary.

Barton had sailed on the USS *Essex* to Europe in 1810 and toured navy medical facilities in Great Britain and France. Upon his return, he brought to the American navy many of the ideas promoted by British and French naval surgeons, including where to anchor a ship in an unhealthy harbor, avoiding the tropical sun, and proper dress for the climate. Ship construction, he suggested, must include ventilation of the lower decks; to rid the ship of dampness, which he thought caused disease, daily deck scrubbing must be limited and fires lighted between decks to dry the air.

In discussing the health and treatment of seamen, he said the navy should enforce laws for honest and fair treatment and provide them with work fit for a seaman, not working with a shovel and wheelbarrow, which was for landlubbers and deeply resented. It was not uncommon for crew to go on sick call or even desert when ordered to do such tasks.

Barton relates how, when discharged, the typical sailor—his pockets stuffed with discharge pay—says good-bye to his shipmates and heads for the nearest bar; within an hour he is drunk and cursing his shipmates and officers. He has lost all of his pay and is in debt for his lodging and food. Only one recourse is left him, to re-enlist.

Barton's views were very paternalistic. He believed that officers should substitute for the parents of the enlisted men, many of whom were no more than sixteen years of age and sometimes younger. He recommended that payout at discharge should be over an extended time period, not in a lump sum.

Returning from the West Indies, on board the *Brandywine,* he moralized about the evils of alcohol and tobacco and noted that officers and midshipmen who abstained remained healthier. On the other hand, he criticized officers for permitting men to sleep on deck when in harbor, where they would develop disease from the night air.

Barton correctly diagnosed yellow fever and insisted that it was not contagious. In this he was correct, but he went further and denied that any disease was contagious. At that time, there was a medical dispute in America between the contagionists, led by a Dr. Hosack, and the non-contagionists, led by Dr. Benjamin Rush in Philadelphia. Barton defers to Rush, who was the most prominent physician in the United States and whose false doctrines of disease delayed the advance of medicine here.

Barton claimed the contagionist theories to be "an illusive non-tenable doctrine." If disease is spread by contagion, Barton logically asked, why don't the medical officers and the nurses sicken? Referring to yellow fever, not knowing that it depends on the bite of an infected mosquito, he described cases in which the disease struck when a ship anchored before landing, Like Rush, he attributed disease to moisture arising in a cloud from a swampy shoreline or a foul hold.

The naval establishment in which Barton served paid little respect to health issues that were, as they still are, very important to sailors. Shipboard surgeons were commissioned but held no rank until later in the century. They were helpless in the face of many diseases and unable to cope with many injuries. They were often looked down upon and sneered at by line officers, but to the crew the surgeon was a vital necessity in supporting their health, and his presence increased morale in battle.

In the general mutiny of the British fleet at Spithead in England, for instance, the principal grievance was not cruel punishment, long voyages, battle dangers, overwork, and long hours but the neglect of the sick, the embezzlement of medical and general supplies, the lack of the sailor's few comforts, and ignoring his needs for medicines and doctors. The requests of the mutinous crews were addressed to the lords and commissioners of the Admiralty, who accepted their demands.

In his book on the organization and government of marine hospitals, Barton applied himself to the construction and internal organization of such hospitals and goes a step further by proposing the reorganization of the entire medical department of the navy.[18]

Barton recommended lemon juice for scurvy, and to preserve it on a long sea journey he spiked it with brandy, which certainly reduced its potency. No one person in this period in Britain, Europe, or America unequivocally stated that scurvy was prevented and cured by green vegetables or citrus fruit. Salted meats, wet clothing, overwork, and filth were still held to be contributing causes. Even James Lind, whose name is associated with citrus fruits and fresh greens, considered the cause of scurvy to be multifactoral.

There was still no specific directive concerning scurvy in the American navy, although the British Admiralty finally yielded in 1795 and mandated lemon juice to all personnel after fourteen days at sea. In America each surgeon and captain decided what measures to take. The USS *President* was forced to curtail her tour of duty in 1812, after only four weeks at sea, because of an outbreak of scurvy. Other vessels were also out of action for this reason. The American frigate *Macedonian* in 1827 had an especially bad experience, losing 101 men of a crew of 376 from scurvy.[19] With the information available at that time about scurvy, such a catastrophe warranted a court-martial of the surgeon and captain.

In 1811 Congress allowed the navy to have its own hospitals in the United States to improve the health of navy personnel. Congress had already enacted legislation to provide health care for the crews of the merchant marine. Barton wanted all surgeons in the navy to be medical school graduates, although he allowed surgeon's mates to be apprentice trained (thus without any chances of advancement unless they went to medical school). The instruments and medications brought on board by the surgeons were to be officially prescribed and not of the doctor's choosing.

There was at that time no rank given a surgeon in the U.S. Navy, although in the British military a surgeon's rank in the navy was a lieutenant and equivalent to the army rank of captain. The American surgeon was to receive fifty dollars a month plus two rations a day; the surgeon's mate received thirty dollars a month, with two rations.

William Crillon Barton, the upstart surgeon so disdainful of his superiors, who ruffled the navy brass, was made chief of the Bureau of Medicine of the Navy in 1842. In a tour of Britain and France, he spent time at naval hospitals and studied shipboard medicine and medical practices in both countries and then transposed the teachings of leading authorities across the Atlantic to America. In particular, he absorbed the views of the eminent British naval surgeons Trotter, Blane, and Lind, which he applied to the American navy. Lime juice was emphasized for scurvy, and shipboard cleanliness to avoid disease. The navy hospitals were reorganized, the duties of the surgeon reclarified, and the working conditions of the crew improved.[20] After resigning from the Navy, Barton became professor of botany at the University of Pennsylvania.

Reliance on Medical Manuals

American merchant vessels sailing in all the seas of the world sometimes carried a surgeon, but most did not. Scores of whaling vessels left New England ports each year for extended voyages of two to three years, engaged in the dangerous game of killing and rendering of whales, without a doctor. Usually the captain or a designated officer assumed the role of doctor, and with little or no training had to make life-and-death decisions after an injury. Wives of officers often accompanied them and were helpful as nurses. (Children, however, were another problem.)

During long voyages, the men's lack of outside contacts protected them from disease, but upon landfall they were subject to smallpox, cholera, dysentery, malaria, yellow fever, measles, and bubonic plague. Disease could rage throughout the vessel.

In the captain's cabin of American merchant ships, a medical guide book was second in importance only to the tables of navigation and charts. An early and popular medical book was *The Planters and Mariners Medical Companion* by John Ewell, published in 1807, which was dedicated to Thomas Jefferson. Later, Usher Parsons, the naval surgeon and hero of the Battle of Lake Erie, wrote the *Sailor's Physician*. These books listed symptoms and recommended prescriptions to overcome the presenting problem. Sometimes they gave information on how to diagnose a specific condition and treat the disease. If the sailor was suffering from diarrhea, the captain could look it up in the index and find pages telling how to compound prescriptions to cure this condition. There were chapters on fevers, pleurisy, earache, nosebleeds, epilepsy, fractures, dislocations, and wounds and how to deliver a baby.[21]

For the officer acting as accoucheur, it wisely suggested to allow nature to proceed and not to interfere with the delivery. To avoid sepsis, the cabin was to be scrupulously cleansed and properly ventilated to avoid the accumulation of toxic air. The mother was to be confined in a horizontal position, and proper timing and tying of the umbilical cord was detailed. Complaints and treatment of women's and children's diseases were also itemized.

In the United States in 1790, a law mandated that every vessel carry a medicine chest provided by a competent apothecary and accompanied by a medical manual. Such a chest would contain opium for pain relief, quinine or cinchona bark for fevers, mercury compounds for venereal disease (also used as a cathartic), ipecac, castor oil, ointments, lotions, and weight scales and measures, as well as a mortar and pestle.

For surgery, bandages and splints were stocked as well as catheters, syringes, and a small knife for bleeding; larger knives for making incisions and amputation knives and saws, in addition to needles and thread for closing wounds, were listed.

The responsibility for such medical decisions must have weighed heavily on the shoulders of the officer selected to serve in the doctor's role, and the ship's course was often altered if a doctor could be found in an accessible shore community.[22]

The War of 1812

In 1812, the U.S. Navy was once again tested in defending the commerce of the nation, this time against British seizures. President Madison signed a declaration of war against the British on 18 June 1812. The six frigates launched in 1797 and 1798 formed the nucleus of the navy. Nineteen vessels in all constituted the fleet, which consisted of seven frigates, nine schooners and brigs, and three unserviceable vessels. Each ship in service carried one surgeon and one or two surgical mates.

It was reckoned that, with the new ships being added to the fleet, forty-four surgeons and forty-six mates would be called to the colors. Recruiting for surgeons was the responsibility of the ship commanders, just as it was in the army. Most surgeons who volunteered were trained as apprentices, did not have a medical degree, and were often at sea for as long as a year before their commissions were granted. This system of procurement proved so unsatisfactory that in 1825 a board of surgeons started granting commissions only upon the candidates' passing an examination.

Congress, in 1811, had authorized a hospital for naval personnel, but it was not yet ready to serve the casualties of the War of 1812. Those naval casualties who returned to port were treated in the homes of private families and attended by community physicians. The treasury paid two dollars and fifty cents to three dollars a week for board and paid the bills of the local physicians. Some naval personnel also convalesced in the merchant marine hospitals in Boston, Philadelphia, and New York and the Charity Hospital in New Orleans.

Dress regulations for surgeons issued at this time included a blue coat with broad lapels and a standing collar, with a double row of gold buttons embossed with a frog. A white vest and breeches and a cocked hat completed the uniform. Surgical mates had the same uniform, without the gold buttons. The loblolly boys (corpsmen), like other seamen, wore what they wanted.

Amos Alexander Evans served an apprenticeship with several doctors, including Dr. Benjamin Rush of Philadelphia. Evans joined the navy as a surgeon's mate in 1808 but, being dissatisfied with his position as a surgeon's mate, took time off and was granted a medical degree from Harvard before returning to the navy. In 1812, he was appointed to the frigate *Constitution* after war had been declared against Britain. He sailed from Washington on 11 June 1812 and kept a detailed journal of his activities.

Evans had a deep love for the sea and ecstatically described in his log his delight on walking the spar deck and gazing upward at the mass of rigging stretching skyward as great clouds of canvas billowed in the breeze, the deck pitching as the bow knifed through the Atlantic swells.

> August 19, 1812. Course SW., wind N by E, Latitude observed 41° 42' N, Longitude by D.R. 55° W. At 2 P.M. discovered a large sail to leeward. Made sail and stood down for her. At 4 P.M. discovered her to be a large frigate. When we were within two and a half miles, she hoisted English Colours and fired a gun. . . . We hoisted our colours and fired the first gun about five minutes past 5 P.M., but did not come into close action until about 6 o'clock, and after twenty five minutes from this time we were closely engaged, she struck, having previously lost all three of her masts and the bowsprit.

After this the *Guerriere* floated helplessly. Surrender of a ship usually was the result of destroying her maneuverability, an uncontrolled fire on board, or explosion of her powder magazine. High casualties might force surrender, too. The *Guerriere* had fifteen killed and sixty-two wounded, many of them seriously. The *Constitution's* losses were seven killed and eight wounded. Most of the enemy's casualties were from grape and canister shot.

> Assisted Dr. Irwin, Surgeon of the *Guerriere* to dress his wounded, and amputated two arms and one thigh. Then amputated the leg of Rich Dunn. Had no sleep all night dressing wounded men as they came on board. . . . [After all of the crew of the *Guerriere* was removed and on board the *Constitution*] . . . we set her on fire. Our ship with the boat she blew up presenting a sight, the most incomparably grand and magnificent, I have ever experienced. No poet or painter or historian could give on canvas or paper any description that would do justice to the scene.[23]

James Inderwyck

There were, of course, defeats as well. Dr. James Inderwyck was appointed surgeon on the brig *Argus,* which left for France carrying American diplomats. Inderwyck graduated from Columbia College in 1808. Later he went to medical school for one year and may have taken courses at other schools also. He was appointed house surgeon at New York Hospital between 1812 and 1813.

On 11 May 1813, he sailed on the *Argus,* whose orders were to disrupt British shipping after delivering American diplomats to France. She very effectively carried out this part of her mission, destroying a large number of merchantmen off the southwest coast of Britain. She was known to mariners in Britain as the "Phantom Ship," and her plundering raised insurance rates to such heights that owners feared to sail their ships in the area and protested to the government. The Admiralty ordered warships to track and destroy her.

In his journal, Inderwyck described the battle between the *Argus* and the brig HMS *Pelican* off the coast of Ireland on 14 August 1813. The battle began at 6:00 A.M. At 6:04, Captain Allen of the *Argus* was sent below with a shattered knee. At 6:12 the *Argus's* first mate, Watson, suffered a scalp wound and was sent to the cockpit.

By 6:18 the *Argus* had lost the use of her after sails and was unmanageable, and by 6:30, when the first mate returned to the deck, the *Pelican* was again astern and within pistol shot. Seventeen minutes later, according to the doctor, Watson surrendered *Argus* as the British prepared to board her. When the smoke cleared the British flag was seen flying over the American frigate and both vessels were lying broadside two hundred yards apart, making emergency repairs. It was then Inderwyck's turn. While Watson took command, the surgeon amputated Captain Allen's leg through the mid-thigh. Later Inderwyck dressed Watson's wound.

Casualties on the *Argus* were eight killed and ten wounded. On the *Pelican,* two were killed and five wounded.

The casualties other than Captain Allen were listed by Inderwyck. There were three gunshot wounds of the femur, but no additional amputations for femoral gunshot wounds. One wounded man died. Of two leg wounds, one was amputated and the other refused amputation. We have no record of any follow-up. In addition, Inderwyck treated wounded with a laceration of the chest, a calf laceration, a thigh laceration, a wound of the eye, and a back injury, all of whom lived.

Inderwyck reported in his log that Captain Allen's stump was in a good state on 17 August and that he was transferred to the military prison hospital in Plymouth. The following day, he continued treatment and reported the captain as restless and vomiting; the stump was discharging a thin fluid with the appearance of "a want of action of parts." His skin was cold, pulse feeble; a delirium and coma were soon followed by death. Infection and sepsis had claimed the captain.

On Saturday, 21 August 1813, eight British captains were Captain Allen's pallbearers, carrying his coffin, draped by an American ensign on top of which lay his hat and sword. In 1815, Dr. Inderwyck was surgeon on the *Epervier* when it was lost at sea with all hands.[24]

David Glasgow Farragut

A most vivid description of medical care aboard a frigate while engaged in battle is told in the diary of a twelve-year-old midshipman aboard the U.S. frigate *Essex*. David Glasgow Farragut was the captain's aide as the *Essex* dueled with the British frigates *Phoebe* and *Cherub* in the War of 1812 in waters of the Pacific, just off the coast of Valparaiso, Chile, far removed from the usual Atlantic and Caribbean battle zones.

David was alternatively quarter gunner, powder boy, and captain's messenger, observing and recording the maelstrom of the battle. Running across the deck, he stopped in his tracks as the boatswain's mate standing near him was struck by a cannon ball that mutilated and killed him. Horrified at seeing death for the first time, he sickened and sobbed. Yet in the next few minutes the death of so many of his comrades became commonplace and he accommodated to the sight of death and injury.

It was shortly afterward that a midshipman named Isaacs came to the captain and reported that quartergunner Roach had deserted his position. The only reply from the captain was addressed to David: "Do your duty, sir."

The boy's diary read, "I seized a pistol and went in pursuit of the fellow, but didn't find him." Within the space of thirty minutes after he had stood shocked at viewing his first death, he had been ordered to be an executioner. Later, he reflected about the character of Roach. When the battle was going in favor of the *Essex,* Farragut had seen Roach in an exposed position, sleeves rolled up, cutlass in hand, ready to board the enemy, but when the tide of battle reversed, he left his post. Roach was brave with a prospect of victory, but a coward in adversity.

After the *Essex* struck her colors, and the guns were silent, David went below, and on seeing the heaps of mangled bodies of his shipmates dying, "with the most patriotic sentiments on their lips," a wave of horror overcame him as he became faint and sick.

> As soon as I recovered from my shock however, I hastened to assist the surgeon in staunching and dressing the wounds of my comrades. The cockpit, steerage, ward room and berths were filled with wounded. Among the badly wounded was my best friend Lieutenant J. G. Cowell. When I spoke to him he said, "Oh, Davey, I fear it is all up with me." I found that he had lost a leg just above the knee, and the Doctor informed me that his life might have been saved if he consented to the amputation an hour before; but when it was proposed to drop another patient to attend to him he replied, "No Doctor, none of that; fair play is a jewel."
>
> Many of our fine fellows died for want of a tourniquet.

Doctors Hoffman and Montgomery, his mate, escaped unhurt, although some patients were killed by flying splinters while being attended. "These gentlemen exhibited great skill and nerve in their care of the wounded," David wrote, and he wondered at the tenacity of the wounded to live. "It is astonishing what powers of endurance some men possess. There was one man who swam to shore (a mile away) with scarcely one inch of his body that was not burned. . . . Another swam to shore with part of the barrel of a cannon in his flesh."

David Farragut himself had courage in great quantity. As a prisoner aboard the *Phoebe,* he was sent to the steerage and was aroused from his tears and dejection by the cry of a British sailor, "A prize!"

> I saw at once that he had under his arm a pet pig belonging to our ship called, "Murphy." I claimed the animal as my own.
>
> "Ah," said they, "but you are a prisoner and your pig also."
>
> "We always respect private property," I replied as I seized hold of Murphy and determined not to let go unless compelled by superior force. This was fun for the oldsters who immediately sung out, "Go it, my little Yankee! If you can thrash Shorty, you shall have your pig."
>
> "Agreed," said I.
>
> A ring was formed in the open space and at it we went. I soon found that my opponent's pugilistic education did not come up to mine. In fact, he was no match for me, and was compelled to give up the pig. So I took master Murphy under my arm, feeling that I had in some degree wiped out the disgrace of our defeat.

The casualties of the *Essex* included fifty-eight killed, thirty-nine severely wounded, twenty-seven slightly wounded, and thirty-one who were missing. Most of the missing were drowned. The *Phoebe's* loss was four killed and seven wounded. The *Essex* wounded were transported to a house on shore, and treatment was continued there by the surgeon, Dr. Richard Hoffman, assisted by his mate, Dr. Alexander Montgomery, and D. P. Adams, the chaplain, and Midshipman David Farragut, who worked long hours for many days rolling bandages, dressing the wounded, and doing general nursing. David later remarked, "I never earned Uncle Sam's money so faithfully as I did during that hospital service."

The U.S. Navy, in common with the customs of the new republic, abhorred any suggestion of titles or special privileges, so the rank of admiral did not exist when this boy served on the *Essex.* David Glasgow Farragut continued his naval career, was the hero of the battle of Mobile Bay in the Civil War, and became the first officer given the rank of admiral in the U.S. Navy.

There are several aspects of this account that merit further comment. The surgeons were at fault if men died for lack of a tourniquet. Blane, surgeon under Rodney in the Caribbean, wrote of the necessity of providing tourniquets and instructed the wounded to keep a loosened tourniquet around their injured limb, to be tightened if needed. Blane carried a pocket full of tourniquets during battle, and his writings were well known to

American medical officers. Additional seamen should have been assigned to the doctors to transport the wounded and for general assistance. If a triage system had been in effect, the wounds of Lieutenant Cowell would have demanded first priority, and he should have had his amputation at the proper time.

The great discrepancy of casualties between the *Essex* and the *Phoebe* must reflect on seamanship. Captain Hilyar of the *Phoebe* played a cat-and-mouse game with Porter, the captain of the *Essex,* refusing to commence battle until he had the undisputed advantage of position and the wind. Farragut in a later report criticized the tactics of the battle.[25]

Usher Parsons

In September 1813, an American naval squadron under Commodore Perry triumphed over a British squadron commanded by Captain Barclay on Lake Erie. This battle firmly established the new nation as a sea power, recognized by the international community. Two heroes emerged from this engagement. Perry, who led the American squadron to victory over Britain at the zenith of her mastery of the seas, was one. The other hero, not so well known, was surgeon's mate Usher Parsons, on the American flagship *Laurence.* There were three surgeons in Perry's fleet, but two of them were seriously sick, so that all of the care of the American casualties was the responsibility of Parsons, who later published his experience in the *New England Journal of Medicine* in 1818.[26]

The nine vessels of the United States fleet, with six hundred officers and men, left port in good health, but two days out of port an epidemic of a bilious remittent fever spread throughout the vessels. Fortunately, it was quickly overcome and resulted in only one death. This was not typhus, but some intestinal infection.

As the fleets approached, the grog ration was brought out and the fife and drum struck up "all hands to quarters." The ships were of shallow draft and there was no cockpit, so the surgeon used the wardroom as his dressing station and operating room. All hatches were closed at the onset of battle except one, to allow light into the wardroom. Commodore Perry assigned six men to take the wounded below. At noon the battle started, and within minutes casualties were brought below. The *Laurence* was badly mauled. Perry kept calling down to Parsons to send up his assistants for deck duty; after the seventh such call, Parsons told Perry that he no longer had any assistants. The wounded were brought down faster than he could attend them, and he spent all of his time stanching active bleeding and putting splints on broken limbs. With no space left in the wardroom, he dragged the wounded to an adjacent cabin. Missiles penetrated the deck and struck the wounded being treated. He recalled, "Midshipman Lamb came down with his arm badly fractured; I applied a splint and requested he go forward and while my hand was on him, a cannon ball struck on the side and dashed him across the other side of the room which instantly terminated his suffering."

Parsons counted six cannon shots passing through his workplace. As he worked in the dim light, the firing guns and the rumbling of the gun carriages on the deck above him made it impossible to talk to his patients. Blood from the deck seeped into his dressing station. The action lasted until three o'clock, when the British surrendered.

When the firing ceased, Parsons went to work with renewed energy and by nightfall all active bleeding was under control Being the only medical officer and having worked without interruption for six hours, he elected not to begin the amputations without any assistance and without any light. Instead he dispensed opiates and adjusted splints for the remainder of the night.

At daybreak he started his first amputation, and continued until 11:00 A.M. when the last patient was removed from the ward room. Then he turned his attention to dislocations, lacerations, fractures, and penetrating wounds, working until midnight.

The next morning he was rowed over to the *Niagara* to assess the casualties and arranged to have them transported to the *Laurence*, which was now a hospital ship. Through the day he treated the wounded of the *Niagara* and the other vessels. That evening he began to treat the sick.

Ninety-six men were wounded, presenting with twenty-five open fractures, three closed fractures, thirty-seven penetrating wounds, in addition to cerebral, chest, and pelvic injuries. Remarkably, only three of his postoperative patients died.

In evaluating his results, Parsons noted that fractures healed slowly because the motion of the ship in rough weather caused redisplacement of the bones in their splints. He also noted that the delay in attending to the amputations did not impair the healing, and he attributed the rapid healing of his wounded to the purity of the sea air. He brought his patients out of the hold and arranged them on deck under an awning for two weeks before they were brought ashore and received an abundance of fresh food contributed by Ohio farmers. Lastly, Parsons was convinced that the euphoria of victory was in itself beneficial for healing, and that the conquering side will be more successful in wound healing than the vanquished.

Captain Barclay, the British commander, was court-martialed after his defeat by the Americans, but the testimony of the court showed he fought competently and bravely and he was acquitted. The Lords of the Admiralty were forced to accept the naval prowess of the United States with grudging admiration.

Perry wrote to the secretary of the navy, "Of Dr. Usher Parsons, surgeon's mate, I cannot say too much. In consequence of the disability of both other surgeons . . . the whole duty of dressing, operating and attending nearly a hundred wounded, and as many sick developed entirely on him. . . . I can only say that in the event of my having another command, I should consider myself particularly fortunate in having him with me as surgeon."

Parsons received a medal from Congress and $1,214.29 as his share of the prize money due him for his part in the capture of the British fleet. In 1817 he went back to school and received his M.D. degree from Harvard.[27]

* * *

The War of 1812 ended an epoch that extended back into history for more than two hundred years. It saw the last naval battle in which wooden, unarmored sailing vessels confronted each other, broadside to broadside, pouring in cannon fire at close range, raking the decks with devastating effect. Armored wooden vessels, closely followed by steel ships powered by steam, were on the horizon.

In medicine and surgery, too, new ideas were displacing the old beliefs. The notion of a single universal illness, curable by a common drug, could no longer be sustained. Each disease and its cure was a study in itself and required long and painstaking efforts to be unraveled and understood. The process of reaching such understanding was to be experimental science. Doctors had learned by experience how to palliate most infectious diseases but were unable to effect a cure.

The discovery of anesthesia allowed deliberate surgical reconstructions, replacing the hasty, slashing scramble to incise and explore the wound and salvage the wounded. Surgeons of this period were well trained in anatomy, and they understood the rudiments of wound healing, but had no knowledge of microscopic pathology and bacteriology, and only basic pharmacology.

Credit is due those sea surgeons working in the dim light of the cockpit whose spirit, courage, and diligence gave them the strength to cure the sick and injured in spite of their lack of modern medical knowledge.

Notes

Chapter 1. The Origins of Naval Medicine

1. William L. Mann, "The Origin and Early Development of Naval Medicine," 772–82 (1929).

2. William R. Smart, "On the Medical Services of the Navy from the Accession of Henry VIII to the Restoration," *British Medical Journal* (7 February 1874): 264–66.

3. Ibid.

4. John Keevil, *Medicine in the Navy*, vol. 1 (London: E. & S. Livingstone, 1957), 149.

5. John Woodall, *The Surgeon's Mate* (1655).

6. L. H. Roddis, *A Short History of Nautical Medicine* (New York: Paul Hoeber, 1941).

7. Christopher Lloyd and John Coulter, *Medicine in the Navy*, vol. 3 (London: E. & S. Livingstone, 1961).

8. Ibid. 11.

9. Ibid., 10, 33.

10. Ibid., 58.

11. Ibid., 14.

12. Charles N. Robinson, "Notes on the Dress of British Seamen," *Mariner's Mirror* 3, no. 6 (June 1913): 174.

13. Robert Robertson, *Observations on the Diseases of Seamen* (1804).

Chapter 2. Practicing Medicine at Sea

1. John Woodall, *A Treatise on Gangrene and Sphacelos* (1653); *Viaticum* (1653; originally written in 1626); *A Treatise on the Plague* (1653); *The Surgeon's Mate* (1655).

2. John Lind, *An Essay on the Health of Seamen* (1774).

3. Woodall, *Treatise on the Plague*.

4. John Keevil, *Medicine in the Navy*, vol. 1 (London & Edinburgh: E. & S. Livingstone, 1957).

5. S. J. Glass, "James Lind, M.D.: Eighteenth Century Naval Hygienist," *Journal of the Royal Navy Medical Service* 34, no. 5 (1948–49): 75–90.

6. Sir Francis Drake, *A Full Relation of Another Voyage to the West Indies made by Sir Francis Drake, Sir John Hawkins and others Being Set Forth on the 28th of August, 1595* (1652).

7. Ibid.

8. Ibid.

9. Baron Van Swieten, quoted by William Northcote in *The Diseases Incident to the Armies* (Philadelphia: R. Bell, 1776). This book draws extensively from Van Swieten's *Marine Practice of Physic and Surgery.*

10. Lloyd and Coulter, *Medicine in the Navy*, vol. 3 (London & Edinburgh: E. & S. Livingstone, 1961).

11. Robert Young, *Surgeon's Journal*, ADM 101/85. PRO.

12. Gilbert Blane, *Observations on the Diseases of Seamen* (1789).

13. Tobias Smollett, *Roderick Ransom* (1748).

14. Thomas Ritter, *Medicine Chest Companion on Shipboard* (1866).

15. Eleanora Gordon, "The Captain as Healer: Medical Care on Merchantmen and Whalers," *American Neptune* 54, no. 4 (Fall 1994): 265–77.

16. Ibid.

17. Samuel Samuels, *From the Forecastle to the Cabin on the Famous Packet Ship, Dreadnaught* (1926), 292.

18. John Henry Plumridge, *Hospital Ships and Hospital Trains* (1975), 13.

19. William L. Mann, "The Origin and Early Development of Naval Medicine," U.S. Naval Institute *Proceedings* 55 (September 1929): 772–82.

20. John Stewart, "Hospital Ships in the Second Dutch War," *Journal of the Royal Navy Medical Service* 34 (1948): 29–35.

21. Ibid.

22. Guenter Risse, "Hospital Ships," *History of Medical and Allied Sciences* 43 (1988): 426–46.

23. Plumridge, *Hospital Ships and Hospital Trains*, 14.

24. John Sutherland, "The Hospital Ship, 1608–1740," *Mariner's Mirror* 22, no. 4 (October 1936): 422–26.

25. John Glass, "James Lind, Eighteenth Century Medical Hygienist," *Royal Navy Medical Service* 34–35 (1948–49): 422–26.

26. Sutherland, "The Hospital Ship."

27. Robert Robertson, *Observations on the Diseases of Seamen* (1804).

28. Thomas Trotter, *Medica Nautica*, vol. 3 (London: Longmans, Hurst and Rees, 1804).

29. John Milne, *Diseases That Prevailed in Two Voyages in the Carnatic, East Indiaman (1793–98); Observations in a Series of Letters to John Hunter* (1803).

30. Ibid.

Chapter 3. Battling Disease at Sea

1. Gilbert Blane, *Observations on the Diseases of Seamen* (1789).

2. Samuel Dutton, *A Historical Account of a New Method of Extraction of Air out of Ships* (1749).

3. Trotter, *Medica Nautica* (1804).

4. Robert Robertson, *Observations on the Diseases of Seamen* (1804).

5. Trotter, *Medica Nautica.*

6. Gordon Pugh, *Nelson and His Surgeons* (London & Edinburgh: E. & S. Livingstone, 1968).

7. Christopher Lloyd and John Coulter, *Medicine in the Navy,* vol. 3 (London & Edinburgh: E. & S. Livingstone, 1961).

8. John Keevil, *Medicine in the Navy,* vol. 1 (London & Edinburgh: E. & S. Livingstone, 1957).

9. Richard Allison, *Sea Diseases* (London: John Bale Medical Publications, 1943), 15.

Chapter 4. Scurvy

1. John Freind, M.D., *History of Physick from the Time of Galen to the Sixteenth Century* (1726).

2. Richard Allison, *Sea Diseases* (London: John Bale Medical Publications, 1943), 15.

3. Julian DeZulueta and Lola Higueras, "Health and Navigation in the South Seas," in *Starving Sailors,* ed. Watts, Freeman, and Bynum (Greenwich: National Maritime Museum, 1981).

4. David McBride, *Essays on Medical and Philosophical Subjects* (London: Millar and Caddell, 1767).

5. Christopher Lloyd, "The Influence of Nutrition upon Naval and Maritime History," in *Starving Sailors,* ed. Watts, Freeman, and Bynum (Greenwich: National Maritime Museum, 1981).

6. Edward Arber, *An English Garner: Voyages and Travels* (New York: E. Dutton, 1902).

7. John Woodall, *Viaticum.* Woodall was powerful enough to request of the king a wage increase for the fleet surgeons from 19 shillings 4 pence to 30 shillings, to which Charles agreed. The king also agreed to his request to provide instrument chests for his surgeons and, because of Woodall's influence, gave the Company of Barber-Surgeons a new charter. Additional special gifts were grant-

ed to those surgeons serving on the eighteen great ships of the first rank—the *Triumph, Ange Royall, Saint Andrew, Nonesuch, Unicorne, Swiftsure, Red Lyon, Reformation,* and others—in a ceremony held on the tenth of July, 1626.

8. John Woodall, *The Surgeon's Mate* (1655).

9. Ibid.

10. Richard Hakluyt, *The Principal Navigations, Voyages, Traffiques and Discoveries of the English Nation* (1598).

11. Allison, *Sea Diseases* (London: John Bale Medical Publications, 1943), 28.

12. Julian DeZulueta, "Health in the Spanish Navy during the Age of Nelson," paper presented at the Conference on Health in the Royal Navy, Institute of Naval Medicine, Alverstoke, 1 July 2000.

13. John Clark, *Observations on the Diseases of Long Voyages* (1778).

14. Mead, *A Discourse on Scurvy* (1749); Allison, *Sea Diseases,* 28.

15. Richard Mead, *A Discourse on Scurvy.*

16. Allison, *Sea Diseases,* 102.

17. James Lind, *The Health of Seamen* (1774).

18. David McBride, *Essays on Medical and Philosophical Subjects* (1767).

19. William Hunter, *Essay on the Diseases Incident to Indian Seamen* (Calcutta: The Honourable Company, 1804).

20. James Lind, *Most Effectual Means of Preserving Health of Seamen* (London, 1757).

21. Christopher Lloyd, ed., *The Health of Seamen,* vol. 107, a publication of the Navy Records Society (London & Colchester: Spottiswoode, Ballantyne and Co. Ltd., 1965).

22. John Milne, *Diseases That Prevailed in Two Voyages to the East Indies in the Carnatic East Indiaman During Years of 1763–68* (London: E. Spraggs, 1803). The penurious young surgeon, forced to live aboard the *Carnatic* while she was still being provisioned in the harbor, made some interesting observations. Custom permitted ladies from the town of Gravesend to come aboard, and the surgeon was soon treating numerous members of the crew for venereal disease (known to accentuate the symptoms of scurvy). Milne also described a ploy practiced by crewmembers who were given a bounty and two months' wages for signing on. When the ship anchored again at Portsmouth, just prior to departure from the country, a rowboat would stealthily advance toward the ship and tie up under the bowsprit. Crew members jumped ship to the rowboat and went ashore, to repeat the process with the next departing ship.

23. Lloyd, ed., *The Health of Seamen,* 107: 298.

24. James Lind, *Treatise of Scurvy* (1753); *Essay on the Most Effectual Means of Preserving the Health of Seamen* (1754).

25. James Lind, *Dissertations on Fevers and Infections* (London: Wilson, 1757).

26. J. Glass, "James Lind, Eighteenth Century Naval Hygienist," *Journal of the Royal Navy Medical Service* 34–35 (1948–49): 3–20.

27. Thomas Trotter, *Observations on the Scurvy* (1786).

28. Lloyd, ed., *The Health of Seamen.*

29. Trotter, *Observations on the Scurvy.*

30. Lloyd, ed., *The Health of Seamen.*

31. Ibid.

32. Allison, *Sea Diseases,* 144.

33. *Philosophical Transactions of the Royal Society,* vol. 16, part 1 (1776).

34. Sir James Watts, "Medical Aspects and Consequences of Cook's Voyages," in *Captain Cook and His Times,* ed. Robin Fraser and Hugh Johnston (Seattle: University of Washington Press, 1979).

35. K. Diem and C. Lentner, *Scientific Tables* (Basle: Ciba-Geigy, 1970).

36. DeZulueta and Higueras, "Health and Navigation in the South Seas."

37. Adrien Carré, "Eighteenth Century French Voyages of Exploration," in *Starving Sailors,* ed. Watts, Freeman, and Bynum (Greenwich: National Maritime Museum, 1981).

38. The carronade gun was a short-barreled, lightweight gun like a mortar, firing a heavy shot for a short distance; it was also called a "smasher."

39. Hakluyt, *Traffiques and Discoveries.*

Chapter 5. Beriberi

1. Arthur Bentley, *Beriberi* (1893); Edward Vedder, *Beriberi* (New York: William Wood & Co., 1913), 54, 59.

2. William Hunter, *An Essay on the Diseases Incident to Indian Seamen or Lascars on Long Voyages* (1804).

3. Ibid.

4. Selene Yeager, *The Doctors' Book of Food Remedies* (Rodale, 1997), 74.

5. Hunter, *Diseases Incident to Indian Seamen.*

6. Ibid.

7. Ibid.

8. Duane Simmons, Report printed by Inspector General of Customs, Shanghai, 1880.

9. Andrew Davidson, "Beriberi," in *Manson's Hygiene and Diseases of Warm Climates* (1893).

Chapter 6. Typhus and Tropical Fevers

1. Richard Allison, *Sea Diseases* (London: John Bale Medical Publications Ltd., 1943).

2. James Lind, *The Most Effectual Means of Preserving the Health of Seamen* (1757).

3. Ibid.

4. Robert Robertson, *Observations on the Diseases of Seamen* (1804).

5. Carlo Cogressi, "New Theory of Contagious Disease Among Oxen," paper presented at the Seizone Lombarda della Società Italia di Microbiologica (Rome, 1953), 17.

6. John Keevil, *Medicine in the Navy*, vol. 1 (London & Edinburgh: E. & S. Livingstone, 1957), 159.

7. John Spinney, "Fumigation of Ships," *Mariner's Mirror* 150 (February 1964): 282.

8. James Lind, *Most Effectual Means*.

9. Ibid.

10. John Hunter, *Diseases of the Army in Jamaica*, 3rd ed. (1808).

11. William Baldwin, *A Short Narrative of the Diseases Which Prevailed among the American Seamen at Whampoa, China* (1807).

12. John Milne, *Diseases That Prevailed on Two Voyages to the East Indies* (1803).

Chapter 7. Death and Disease in the Slave Trade

1. Anonymous, *A Short Account of That Part of Africa Inhabited by Negroes* (1762).

2. Richard Hakluyt, *The Principal Navigations, Voyages, Traffiques and Discoveries of the English Nation* (1598).

3. Thomas J. Hutchinson, *Hutchinson's West Africa* (1858).

4. Ibid.

5. Alexander Falconbridge, *An Account of the Slave Trade on the Coast of Africa* (1788). Two of the most active kings in this enterprise were called Peppel and Norfolk by English traders.

6. Ibid.

7. Ibid.

8. Thomas Buxton, *The African Slave Trade* (London: John Murray, 1839).

9. Ibid. The detention camps lacked all sanitation, and the death rate from disease was high. Smallpox and dysentery were the foremost killers. In 1831, a severe epidemic of smallpox in an African detention camp killed hundreds.

10. Thomas Perronet, letter dated 3 August 1809, to a friend in Jamaica; original in Brynmor Jones Library, University of Hull, UK.

11. Falconbridge, *An Account of the Slave Trade*.

12. Anonymous, *A Short Account*.

13. Thomas Winterbottom, *An Account of the Natives of Africa* (1803).

14. This and the following anecdotes of slaving operations on the *Ned, Mary, James, Lively,* and *Mme. Pookate* are drawn from *Journals of Surgeons Employed in the Ships Trading to Africa since August 1, 1788,* House of Lords Library, London.

15. Christopher Bowen, *Medical Diary on the Slave Ship, "Lord Stanley"* (1792).

16. Michael Flynn, *The Second Fleet, 1790* (Sydney: Library of Australian History, 1993).

17. Falconbridge, *An Account of the Slave Trade.*

18. Winterbottom, *An Account of the Natives of Africa.*

19. Falconbridge, *An Account of the Slave Trade.*

20. Winterbottom, *An Account of the Natives of Africa.*

21. Thomas Trotter, *Observations on the Scurvy* (London: Charles Elliot, 1786).

22. Equiano, Olaudah, *The Interesting Narrative of the Life of Olaudah Equiano, the African, Written by Himself,* ed. Paul Edwards (London: Heineman, 1967; published by the author in 1789).

23. Falconbridge, *An Account of the Slave Trade.*

24. John Harris, "The Genuine Account of the Dreadful Massacre That Befell Captain Badd and his people on the Ship Marlborough," letter to his father published in *Felix Farley's Bristol Journal,* 24 March 1753.

25. A U.S. Coastal Survey brig intercepted *Amistad* and delivered her to New London, Connecticut. The Africans subsequently pleaded for their freedom in the U.S. courts. Thirty-six of them were eventually repatriated in 1841 through the intervention of abolitionists, as well as the advocacy of John Quincy Adams.

26. George Crowley, letter dated 27 September 1752, to William Pitt. Chatham Papers, Public Record Office 30/8 #708, 58–61 and 208–9, London.

27. Anonymous, *Case of the Vigilante* (1823).

Chapter 8. Impressment and Punishment

1. Christopher Lloyd, *The Health of Seamen* (London: Navy Record Society, 1965).

2. C. S. Forester, ed., *The Diary of John Wetherill* (London: Michael Joseph, 1954).

3. Ibid.

4. Enoch Wines, *Two and a Half Years in the Navy Aboard the U.S. Frigate Constellation* (1832).

5. Tilton, J., *Oeconomical Observations on the Military Hospitals and the Prevention and Cure of Diseases Incident to the Army* (1813).

6. Anonymous Lieutenant, U.S. Navy, *Naval Discipline and Corporal Punishment* (1850).

7. S. J. Glass, "James Lind, Eighteenth Century Naval Hygienist," *Journal of the Royal Navy Medical Service* 34–35 (1948–49).

8. Humphrey Rolleston, *Contributions to Medicine and Biology Research* (New York: Paul Hoeber, 1919).

Chapter 9. Shipwrecks and Survivors

1. William B. Doherty and Dagobert O. Runes, *Lesions in Survivors of Shipwreck* (New York: Philosophical Library, 1943), 647, 681.

2. MacDonald Critchley, *Shipwreck Survivors: A Medical Study* (London: J. & A. Churchill Ltd., 1943, 43.

3. Ibid., 57.

4. Ibid., 65.

5. Ibid., 7.

6. Richard Allison, *Sea Diseases* (London: John Bale Medical Publications, 1943), 141.

7. Doherty and Runes, *Lesions in Survivors of Shipwreck,* 647, 681.

8. Louis Roddis, *A Short History of Nautical Medicine* (New York: Paul Hoeber, 1941), 106.

9. Doherty and Runes, *Lesions in Survivors of Shipwreck.*

10. Critchley, *Shipwreck Survivors.*

11. Richard Walter, *A Voyage Around the World of George Anson* (1748).

12. Charles Neider, ed., *Great Shipwrecks and Castaways* (New York: Harper Bros., 1952), 12.

13. Ibid.

14. Ibid.

15. Archibald Duncan, *Mariner's Chronicle* (1835).

16. Walter, *Voyage Around the World.*

17. Louis Becke and Walter Jeffrey, *Naval Pioneers of Australia* (1899).

18. William Bligh, *A Narrative of the Mutiny on Board H.M.S. Bounty and the Subsequent Voyage from Tofoa in the Friendly Islands to Timor* (1790).

19. C. Foster, *1700 Miles in an Open Boat* (New York: Houghton Mifflin, 1924).

20. Caroline Alexander, *The Endurance* (New York: Alfred Knopf, 1998).

21. Norwich, *Means of Assistance in Cases of Shipwreck* (1825).

22. Richard Lewis, *The Lifeboat and Its Work* (1874).

23. George W. Manley, *An Essay on Preservation of Shipwrecked Persons* (1812).

Chapter 10. Marine Medicine in the United States

1. Maurice Gordon, *Naval and Maritime Medicines during the American Revolution* (Ventnor, N.J.: Ventnor Publishers, 1978), 17.

2. David Syrett, "Living Conditions on the Navy Board's Transports during the American War," *Mariner's Mirror* 55, no. 1 (January 1969): 87.

3. Gordon, *Naval and Maritime Medicines,* 17.

4. John Jones, *Plain Concise, Practical Remarks on the Treatment of Wounds and Fractures to which is added an Appendix on Camp and Military Hospitals* (1776).

5. William Baldwin, *A Short Narrative of the Diseases Which Prevailed among the American Seamen at Whampoa China* (1807).

6. Edward Cutbush, letter to John Baughn, 10 July 1801 (American Philosophical Library, Philadelphia).

7. Ibid.

8. Paul Cushman, "Medicine at the Turn of the Century," *New York State Journal of Medicine* 72 (July–December 1972): 1881–87.

9. Edward Cutbush, *Preserving the Health of Soldiers and Sailors* (1808).

10. J. Worth Estes, "Naval Medicine in the Age of Sail," *Bulletin of the History of Medicine* 56 (1982): 238–53.

11. Robert Hancock, "Pestilence from the Seas and American Quarantine Policy," *American Neptune* 50 (Spring 1990): 54–100.

12. Cutbush, *Preserving the Health of Soldiers and Sailors.*

13. Wines, *Two and a Half Years in the Navy Aboard the U.S. Frigate Constellation* (1832).

14. Cutbush, *Preserving the Health of Soldiers and Sailors.*

15. Judah Paddock, *Narrative of the Shipwreck of the Oswego* (1818).

16. Jonathan Cowdery, *Dr. Cowdery's Journal* (1806).

17. Frank L. Pleadwell and William M. Kerr, "Jonathan Cowdery, Surgeon, United States Navy," *United States Navy Medical Bulletin* 17, no. 1 (1922): 63–89.

18. William C. Barton, *A Treatise on the Internal Organization and Government of Marine Hospitals and the Organization of the Medical Department* (1814).

19. Frank Pleadwell, "William C. Barton, 1786–1856, Surgeon, United States Navy," *Military Surgeon* 46 (March 1920): 241–48.

20. Barton, *A Treatise on the Internal Organization and Government.*

21. James Ewell, *The Planter's and Mariner's Medical Companion* (1807); Usher Parsons, *Sailor's Physician, Exhibiting the Symptoms, Causes and Treatment of Diseases Incident to Seamen in Merchant Vessels* (1820).

22. Ewell, *The Planter's and Mariner's Medical Companion.*

23. Amos E. Evans, "Journal Kept on Board the Frigate Constitution, 1812," *Pennsylvania Magazine of History and Biography,* vol. 19 (1895): 152–69, 374–86. Pamphlet, William D. Sawtell, Lincoln, Mass., 1967.

24. Victor Poltsis, ed., "Journal of Surgeon James Inderwyck," *Bulletin of the New York Public Library* 21, no. 6 (1917): 383–85.

25. David Porter, *Journal of a Cruise Made to the Pacific in the United States Frigate Essex in 1812, 1813, 1814* (1815); Loyall Farragut, *The Life of David Glasgow Farragut* (1879).

26. Usher Parsons, "Surgical Account of the Naval Battle on Lake Erie on the 10th of September, 1813," *New England Journal of Medicine* 27 (1818): 313–16.

27. Paul Cushman, "Usher Parsons, M.D., 1788–1868, *New York State Journal of Medicine* 71 (1972): 1881–87.

Bibliography

Works cited or consulted in the preparation of this book include many, from collections in the United States or Great Britain, that are not in general circulation and are in some cases centuries old. The locations of such works are abbreviated in the bibliographic references.

List of Abbreviations

American Philosophical Library	APL
Bristol Central Library, Bristol, UK	BCL
Brynmor Jones Library, Hull, UK	BJL
College of Physicians, Philadelphia	CP
Free Library of Philadelphia	FLP
House of Lords Library, London	HLL
Independence Seaport Museum, Philadelphia	ISM
Library Company of Philadelphia	LCP
Public Record Office, London	PRO
Royal College of Surgeons Library, London	RCS
Van Pelt Library, University of Pennsylvania	VPL

Alexander, Caroline. *The Endurance*. New York: Knopf, 1998.

Allison, Richard Sydney. *Sea Diseases: The Story of a Great Natural Experiment in Preventive Medicine in the Royal Navy.* London: John Bale Medical Publications Ltd., 1943.

Anonymous. *The Case of the Vigilante*. London: Harvey Darton & Co., 1823. LCP.

Anonymous. *An English Garner: Voyages and Travels.* With introduction by Raymond Beazley. New York: E. P. Dutton, 1902.

Anonymous. *A Short Account of That Part of Africa Inhabited by Negroes.* 2nd ed. Philadelphia: W. Dunlap, 1762. LCP.

Anonymous Lieutenant, U.S. Navy. *Naval Discipline and Corporal Punishment.* Boston: Charles P. C. Moody, 1850. LCP.

Arber, Edward. *An English Garner: Voyages and Travels.* Vol. 3. New York: E. P. Dutton, 1902.

Baldwin, William. *A Short Narrative of the Diseases Which Prevailed among the American Seamen at Whampoa, China.* Philadelphia: T. Stiles, printer, 1807. CP.

Barton, William Crillon. *A Treatise for the Internal Organization and Government of Marine Hospitals in the U.S.* Philadelphia: Edward Parker, 1814. CP.

Becke, Louis, and Walter Jeffrey. *Naval Pioneers of Australia.* London: John Murray, 1899. LCP.

Bentley, Arthur J. *Beriberi.* London: J. Young Pentland, 1893. CP.

Blane, Gilbert. *Observations on the Diseases of Seamen.* London: J. Cooper, printer, 1789. CP.

Bligh, William. *A Narrative of the Mutiny on Board H.M.S. Bounty and the Subsequent Voyage from Tofoa in the Friendly Islands to Timor.* London: George Nichol, 1790. LCP.

Bowen, Christopher. "Medical Diary on the Slave Ship Lord Stanley, 23 March–14 August 1792." RCS.

Buxton, Thomas F. *The African Slave Trade.* London: John Murray, 1839. LCP.

Carré, Adrien. "Eighteenth Century French Voyages of Exploration," in *Starving Sailors,* ed. Sir James Watt, E. J. Freeman, and W. F. Bynum. Papers presented at the 1980 Starving Sailors International Symposium on Nutrition. Greenwich, England: National Maritime Museum, 1981.

Clark, John. Observations on the Diseases of Long Voyages. London: J. Murray, 1778. CP.

Cogressi, Carlo. "New Theory of Contagious Disease Among Oxen." Seizone Lombarda della Società Italie di Microbiologica, 1953.

Cowdery, Jonathan. *Dr. Cowdery's Journal.* Boston: Belcher & Armstrong, 1806. CP.

Critchley, MacDonald. *Shipwreck Survivors: A Medical Study.* London: J. & A. Churchill Ltd., 1943.

Crowley, George. Letter to William Pitt, 27 September 1752. Chatham Papers, 30/8 #708, pp. 58–61 and 208–9. PRO.

Cushman, Paul. "Usher Parsons, M.D. (1788–1868): Naval Surgeon in the Battle of Lake Erie." *New York State Journal of Medicine* 71 (1972): 2891–94.

———. "Amos Evans, Surgeon on the USS *Constitution.*" *New York State Journal of Medicine* 71 (1980): 1881–87.

———. "Medicine at the Turn of the Century." *New York State Journal of Medicine* 82 (1982): 81–84.

Cutbush, Edward. Letter to John Baughn, 10 July 1801, including data from his "thermometrical journal" (16 December 1800 to 12 May 1801). APL.

————. *Preserving the Health of Soldiers and Sailors, with Remarks on Hospitals.* Philadelphia: Thomas Dobson, 1808. CP.

Davidson, Andrew. "Beriberi." In *Manson's Hygiene and Diseases of Warm Climates.* London: J. Young Pentland, 1893. CP.

DeZulueta, Julian. "Health in the Navy at the Time of Nelson." Paper presented at the Conference on Health in the Royal Navy, Institute of Naval Medicine, Alverstoke, July 2000.

———— and Lola Higueras. "Health and Navigation in the South Seas." In *Starving Sailors,* ed. Sir James Watts, E. J. Freeman, and W. F. Bynum. Papers presented at the 1980 Starving Sailors International Symposium on Nutrition. Greenwich, England: National Maritime Museum, 1981.

Doherty, William B., and Dagobert O. Runes. *Lesions in Survivors of Shipwreck.* New York: Philosophical Library, 1943.

Drake, Sir Francis. *A Full Relation of Another Voyage to the West Indies Made by Sir Francis Drake, Sir John Hawkins and Others, Being Set Forth on the 28th of August, 1595.* London: Nicholas Bourne, 1652. VPL.

Duncan, Archibald. *Mariner's Chronicle: Containing the Most Remarkable Disasters at Sea.* London: Durrie & Peck, 1834.

Dutton, Samuel. *A Historical Account of a New Method of Extraction of Air Out of Ships.* London: J. Brindley, printer, 1749. CP.

Edwards, Paul, ed. *The Interesting Narrative of the Life of Olaudah Equiano, the African, Written by Himself.* London: Heineman, 1967. First published by the author in 1789.

Estes, J. Worth. "Naval Medicine in the Age of Sail." *Bulletin of the History of Medicine* 56 (1982): 238–53.

Evans, Amos E. "Journal Kept on Board the Frigate *Constitution,* 1812." *Pennsylvania Magazine of History and Biography,* vol. 19 (1895). Pamphlet reprinted for William D. Sawtell, 1967. ISM.

Ewell, James. *The Planter's and Mariner's Medical Companion.* Philadelphia: John Bioran, 1807. ISM.

Falconbridge, Alexander. *An Account of the Slave Trade on the Coast of Africa.* London: J. Phillips & G. Yard, 1788. LCP.

Farragut, Loyall. *The Life of David Glasgow Farragut.* New York: D. Appleton & Co., 1879. LCP.

Flynn, Michael. *The Second Fleet.* Sydney: Library of Australian History, 1993.

Forester, C. S., ed. *The Diary of John Wetherill.* London: Michael Joseph, 1954.

Foster, Cecil Patrick. *1700 Miles in an Open Boat.* New York: Houghton Mifflin, 1924.

Freind, John. *History of Physick from the Time of Galen to the Sixteenth Century.* London: Walthoe, 1726.

Glass, S. J. "James Lind, M.D.: Eighteenth Century Naval Hygienist." *Journal of the Royal Navy Medical Service* 35, no. 5 (1948–49): 1–20.

Gordon, Eleanora. "The Captain as Healer: Medical Care on Merchantmen and Whalers." *American Neptune* 54, no. 4 (Fall 1994): 265–77.

Gordon, Maurice B. *Naval and Maritime Medicines during the American Revolution.* Ventnor, N.J.: Ventnor Publishers, 1978.

Hakluyt, Richard. *Traffiques and Discoveries of the English Nation* (London: Bishop, Newberie and Barker, 1598), from Kenneth Carpenter, *The History of Scurvy.* Cambridge: Cambridge University Press, 1981.

Hancock, Robert. "Pestilence from the Seas and American Quarantine Policy," *American Neptune* (Spring 1990): 54–100.

Harris, John. "The Genuine Account of the Dreadful Massacre That Befell Captain Badd and His People on the Ship 'Marlborough.'" *Felix Farley's Bristol Journal,* 24 March 1753. BCL.

Hunter, John. *Diseases of the Army in Jamaica.* 3rd ed. London: T. Payne, printer, 1808. CP.

Hunter, William. *An Essay on Diseases Incident to Indian Seamen or Lascars on Long Voyages.* Calcutta: The Honourable Company Press, 1804. CP.

Hutchinson, Thomas J. *Hutchinson's West Africa.* London: Longmans, Brown & Green, 1858. LCP.

Jones, John. *Plain Concise, Practical Remarks on the Treatment of Wounds and Fractures, to which is added an Appendix on Camp and Military Hospitals.* Philadelphia: Robert Bell, printer, 1776. CP.

Journals of Surgeons Employed in the Ships Trading to Africa since August 1, 1788. HLL.

Keevil, John. *Medicine in the Navy.* Vols. 1 and 2. Edinburgh & London: E.& S. Livingstone, 1957.

Lewis, Richard. *The Lifeboat and Its Work.* London: MacMillan Co., 1874. ISM.

Lind, James. Dissertations on Fevers and Infections. London: Wilson, 1757.

———. *An Essay on the Health of Seamen.* London: D. Wilson & G. Nichol, 1774. CP.

———. Essay on the Most Effectual Means of Preserving the Health of Seamen. London: Wilson, 1754.

———. *The Most Effectual Means of Preserving the Health of Seamen.* London, 1757.

———. *A Treatise of Scurvy.* London: A. Millar, printed by Sands, Murray & Cochran, 1753.

Lloyd, Christopher, ed. *The Health of Seamen.* Vol. 107. Publication of the Navy Records Society. London and Colchester: Spottiswoode, Ballantyne and Co., 1965.

———. "The Influence of Nutrition upon Naval and Maritime History." In *Starving Sailors,* ed. Sir James Watt, E. J. Freeman, and W. F. Bynum. Papers presented at the 1980 Starving Sailors International Symposium on Nutrition. Greenwich, England: National Maritime Museum, 1981.

———— and John Coulter. *Medicine in the Navy.* Vols. 3 and 4. London & Edinburgh: E. & S. Livingstone, 1961.

Manley, George W. *Essay on Preservation of Shipwrecked Persons.* London: Longmans, Hurst, Rees, Orme & Brown, 1812. CP.

Mann, William L. "The Origin and Early Development of Naval Medicine." U. S. Naval Institute *Proceedings* 55 (1929): 772–82.

McBride, David. *Essays on Medical and Philosophical Subjects.* London: Millar and Cadell, 1767. CP.

Mead, Richard. *A Discourse on Scurvy.* London: J. Brindley, 1741. CP.

Milne, John. *Diseases That Prevailed in Two Voyages in the Carnatic, East Indiaman (1793–98); Observations in a Series of Letters to John Hunter.* London: E. Spragg, 1803. CP.

Neider, Charles. *Great Shipwrecks and Castaways.* New York: Harper Bros., 1952.

Northcote, William. *The Diseases Incident to the Armies, with the Method of Cure by Baron Van Swieten: Extracts from "The Marine Practice of Physic and Surgery."* Philadelphia: R. Bell, 1776. CP.

Norwich (n.f.n.). *Means of Assistance in Cases of Shipwreck.* London: S. Wilkin, 1825. CP.

Paddock, Judah. *Narrative of the Shipwreck of the Oswego.* New York: Capt. James Riley, 1818. ISM.

Parsons, Usher. *Sailor's Physician: Exhibiting the Symptoms, Causes and Treatment of Diseases Incident to Seamen in Merchant Vessels.* Cambridge, Mass.: Hilliard & Metcalf, 1820.

————. "Surgical Account of the Naval Battle on Lake Erie on the 10th of September, 1813." *New England Journal of Medicine* 27 (1818): 313–16.

Perronet, Thomas. Letter to a friend in Jamaica, 3 August 1809. BJL.

Pleadwell, Frank. "William C. Barton, 1786–1856: Surgeon, United States Navy," *Military Surgeon* 46 (March 1920): 241–48.

———— and W. M. Kerr. "Jonathan Cowdery, Surgeon, United States Navy." *United States Navy Medical Bulletin* 17, no. 1 (1922).

Plumridge, John Henry. *Hospital Ships and Hospital Trains.* London: Seeley, Service & Co., 1975.

Poltsis, Victor, ed. "Journal of Surgeon James Inderwyck." *Bulletin of the New York Public Library* 21, no. 6 (1917): 338–40.

Porter, David. *Journal of a Cruise Made to the Pacific in the United States Frigate Essex in 1812, 1813, 1814.* Lexington, Ky.: Bradford and Inskeep, 1815. LCP.

Pugh, Gordon. *Nelson and His Surgeons.* Edinburgh & London: E. & S. Livingstone, 1968.

Risse, Guenter. "Hospital Ships." *History of Medical and Allied Sciences* 43 (1988): 426–46.

Ritter, Thomas. *Medicine Chest Companion on Shipboard.* New York: John Gray, 1866. ISM.

Robertson, Robert. *Observations on the Diseases of Seamen.* London: Robert Wilke, 1804. CP.

Robinson, Charles N. "Notes on the Dress of British Seamen." *Mariner's Mirror* 3, no. 6 (1913): 174–77.

Roddis, L. H. *A Short History of Nautical Medicine.* New York: Paul Hoeber, 1941.

Rolleston, Humphrey. *Contributions to Medicine and Biology Research.* New York: Paul Hoeber, 1919.

Samuels, Samuel. *From the Forecastle to the Cabin on the Famous Packet Ship, Dreadnaught.* Boston: Charles E. Lauriat, 1926.

Simmons, Duane. Report, "Beriberi, or the Kakke of Japan." Shanghai: Inspector General of Customs, 1880. CP.

Smart, William R. "On the Medical Services of the Navy from the Accession of Henry VIII to the Restoration," *British Medical Journal,* 7 February 1874. CP.

Smollett, Tobias. *Roderick Ransom.* New York: Harper Bros., 1836 (first published in 1748). LCP.

Stewart, John. "Hospital Ships in the Second Dutch War." *Journal of the Royal Navy Medical Service* 34 (1948): 29–35.

Surgeon's Journal, ADM 101/85 (1961). PRO.

Sutherland, John J. "The Hospital Ship, 1608–1740." *Mariner's Mirror* 22, no. 4 (October 1936): 422–26.

Syrett, David. "Living Conditions of the Navy Board's Transports During the American War." *Mariner's Mirror* 55, no. 1 (January 1969).

Tilton, J. *Oeconomical Observations on the Military Hospitals and the Prevention and Cure of Diseases Incident to the Army.* Wilmington, Del.: Wilson, 1813. CP.

Trotter, Thomas. *Observations on the Scurvy.* London: Charles Elliot, 1786. CP.

Vedder, Edward B. *Beriberi.* New York: William Wood & Co., 1913.

Walter, Richard. *A Voyage Around the World of George Anson.* London: John Paul Knapton, 1748. FLP.

Watts, Sir James. "Medical Aspects and Consequences of Cook's Voyages." In *Captain Cook and His Times,* ed. Robin Fraser and Hugh Johnston. Seattle: University of Washington Press, 1979.

Wines, Enoch. *Two and a Half Years in the Navy Aboard the U.S. Frigate Constellation.* Philadelphia: Carey and Leo, 1832. LCP.

Winterbottom, Thomas. *An Account of the Natives of Africa.* London: C. Whittingham, 1803. LCP.

Woodall, John. *Dissertations on Fevers and Infections.* London: Wilson, 1757. CP.

————. *The Most Effectual Means of Preserving the Health of Seamen.* London: 1757. CP.

————. *The Surgeon's Mate.* London: John League, printer, 1655. CP.

————. *Treatise of Scurvy.* London: Sands, Murray & Cochran, printers, for A. Millar, 1753. CP.

————. *Viaticum.* London: John League, printer, for Nicholas Bourne, 1653. (Originally written in 1626.) CP.

Index

ABOUT THE AUTHOR

Zachary B. Friedenberg is a professor of orthopaedic surgery at the University of Pennsylvania. As a clinician-scientist, he has investigated the basic sciences of bone formation and fracture healing, and he is the author of more than seventy articles published in scientific periodicals.

Prior to his teaching, clinical, and research activities, he served as a doctor in a frontline field hospital performing surgery in North Africa, Italy, France, and Germany, and participated in three D-day invasions.

Outside of medicine, his interests have always led him to the sea. A scuba diver since the invention of the self-contained underwater breather, he enjoys underwater photography as well as sailing.

Dr. Friedenberg has written about doctors in Colonial America as well as a narrative about his frontline hospital in World War II.